Public Medical Care

Public Medical Care

PRINCIPLES AND PROBLEMS

Franz Goldmann, M.D.

COLUMBIA UNIVERSITY PRESS · NEW YORK

1945

A WARTIME BOOK: THIS COMPLETE EDITION IS PRODUCED IN FULL COMPLIANCE
WITH THE GOVERNMENT'S REGULATIONS FOR CONSERVING PAPER
AND OTHER ESSENTIAL MATERIALS

COPYRIGHT 1945, COLUMBIA UNIVERSITY PRESS, NEW YORK

Foreign agent: OXFORD UNIVERSITY PRESS, Humphrey Milford, Amen House, London, E.C., 4, England, AND B. I. Building, Nicol Road, Bombay, India

MANUFACTURED IN THE UNITED STATES OF AMERICA

PREFACE

ADEQUATE medical care is a fundamental human right. It is as much a necessity of life as food, shelter, clothing, or education. It is no less indispensable to the well-being of society than to the welfare of the individual. It is an essential component of any program for individual and social security.

In every civilized country efforts have been made to organize facilities and services necessary to prevent, cure, and mitigate illness and to reduce, if not prevent, disability, economic insecurity, and dependency. The development has advanced at widely varying rates of speed. On the whole, steady and impressive progress has been made, particularly during the last decades.

As a result of an arduous process of growth, often through trial and error, there have come into existence a large number and great variety of programs designed to distribute—nay, *democratize*—services for the sick. A systematic classification of all these efforts would be beset with the greatest difficulties were it not for the fact that two principal methods of finance have been used, namely, taxation and insurance. In general the combination of these two principles has been favored as the most promising approach to the goal of social security.

The actual situation differs greatly from country to country due to wide variations in needs and available resources and even more so in social philosophy. One group of countries have placed primary emphasis on the wide application of the contributory principle. They have made social insurance the backbone of their national health program, relegated tax-supported facilities and services to a secondary role, and relied on the efforts of voluntary organizations to provide for essential facilities and services not covered by compulsory insurance schemes.

A second group of countries have used the principle of taxation on a comparatively large scale, primarily for the construction, equipment, and improvement of all essential facilities needed by the population. The costs of operating these institutions, including the costs for personnel, and of services furnished by nongovernmental facilities and health professions in private practice are defrayed mainly by programs of compulsory and voluntary health insurance and only to a smaller degree by tax funds.

A third group of countries have favored the allocation of tax funds for the establishment of selected institutional facilities and for payment of services rendered to designated groups in the population. They have left it largely to voluntary effort to provide certain facilities for the care of the sick, such as general hospitals and treatment centers, and to organize group prepayment plans for medical care. In many instances they have adopted compulsory insurance against industrial accidents as a first step toward an inclusive system of social insurance.

The operation of programs based on the insurance principle has been analyzed and evaluated often and thoroughly. In contrast, few studies have been made of the manner in which the principle of taxation has been applied to the organization of medical care. There are detailed descriptions of selected tax-supported services but there is no composite picture of the whole field.

This book deals with public medical care as a social movement. It is organized in two parts.

The first part attempts to analyze, interpret, and appraise public policy in providing, at public expense, facilities and services for the care of the sick. No effort has been made to present the events in strictly chronological sequence. Nor has the emphasis been placed on a factual review of selected programs of public medical care as they stand. Special needs, socio-economic conditions, and social philosophies in various communities differ too greatly to allow generalization of purely local experience. Instead, this presentation tries to follow those currents of thought which have left a deep mark; to find the common elements in the vast number of developments that have taken place when enthusiasm crystallized into programs; and to trace the guiding principles of organization and administration that have emerged in the process of a piecemeal and, often, haphazard growth.

The second part of this book takes up the problem of planning for clinics, hospitals, and related facilities; for organization of professional services; for payment; and for administration of medical care. It endeavors to show the relative merits of the method of taxation and its potential value to the development of broad programs of health and social security in the future, when the realization of freedom from want will tax the ingenuity of all democratic countries.

PREFACE

Grateful acknowledgments for reading and commenting upon smaller or larger parts of my manuscript are due to many experts in the various fields discussed in this book. I am especially indebted to:

Dean A. Clark, M.D., Chief Medical Officer, Office of Vocational Rehabilitation, Washington, D.C.; Clara E. Councell, Health and Sanitation Division, Office of the Coordinator of Inter-American Affairs, Washington, D.C.; Michael M. Davis, Ph.D., Chairman, Committee on Research in Medical Economics, and Editor, *Medical Care*, New York, N.Y.; James A. Hamilton, Director, New Haven Hospital, and Past President, American Hospital Association, New Haven, Conn.; Samuel W. Hamilton, M.D., Mental Hospital Advisor, United States Public Health Service, Bethesda, Md.; David R. Lyman, M.D., Medical Superintendent, Gaylord Farm Sanatorium, Wallingford, Conn.; Margaret Lovell Plumley, Bureau of Research and Statistics, Social Security Board, Washington, D.C.; Lucille M. Smith, Principal Consultant on Medical Assistance, Bureau of Public Assistance, Social Security Board, Washington, D.C.; Gertrude Sturges, M.D., Consultant on Medical Care, American Public Welfare Association, Chicago, Ill.; C.-E. A. Winslow, Dr. P.H., Professor of Public Health, Yale University School of Medicine, New Haven, Conn.; and Anne Winslow, New York, N.Y.

Many publishers have shown a splendid spirit of cooperation in permitting quotations from their publications. Their names are given in the References under the titles of the works cited.

Above all, I want to thank my wife, Elizabeth Anne. With sympathy and understanding she has assisted me in preparing the manuscript, and with unending patience she has given hundreds of hours to the typewriting and checking of the text.

FRANZ GOLDMANN

New Haven, Conn.
July, 1944

CONTENTS

Part I: Haphazard Growth

1. THE PATTERN OF PROGRESS — 1
2. THE GROWTH OF PUBLIC HOSPITALS — 4
    Facilities for Patients with Communicable Diseases — 8
    Facilities for Patients with Tuberculosis — 16
    Facilities for Patients with Mental Deviations — 22
    General Hospitals — 31
    Unsolved Problems — 42
3. FROM "FREE DISPENSARY" TO PUBLIC MEDICAL CENTER — 43
    Treatment Clinics — 44
    Preventive Clinics — 52
    Private Group Clinics — 61
    The Clinic and the Physician in Private Practice — 63
    Unsolved Problems — 67
4. THE DEVELOPMENT OF PROGRAMS OF PUBLIC MEDICAL CARE FOR "PERSONS IN NEED" — 69
    The Groups Eligible for Public Medical Care — 69
    From the "Paupers" to the "Medically Needy" — 70
    From Emergency Service to Organized Programs — 83
    Professional Services: Organization and Payment — 92
    Care in Clinics, Hospitals, and Custodial Institutions: Organization and Payment — 114
    Administrative Organization — 129
5. ADMINISTRATION OF PUBLIC MEDICAL CARE: ITS PRESENT FRAMEWORK — 151

Part II: Directed Growth

6. PLANNING FOR MEDICAL CARE ... 158
   Planning for Hospitals and Related Facilities ... 160
   Planning for Organization of Professional Services ... 170
   Planning for Payment for Facilities and Services ... 178
   Planning for Administration of Medical Care ... 191
   Underlying Philosophy ... 196

REFERENCES ... 199

INDEX ... 215

> If we could first know where we are and whither we are tending, we could better judge what to do and how to do it.
> ABRAHAM LINCOLN

Part I: Haphazard Growth

· 1 ·

THE PATTERN OF PROGRESS

THE term "public medical care" denotes a special area of community health activities distinguished by two major features: taxation, general or special, is the method by which the funds are obtained; and an agency of government—local, state, or Federal—is responsible for the administration of the service.

This definition, used here in the interest of clear, functional designation of public activities, gives the term public medical care an exact and technical meaning. Not infrequently the word "public" is attached to any nonprofit program or institution offering medical care to groups of people with no regard to the source of funds and the administrative auspices. Such usage reflects the opinion that medical care in general and organized care of the sick in particular is essentially a public service because it benefits the community, serves the common good, and promotes the well-being of society. It visualizes ends to be attained but does not indicate the approach and the methods actually used to accomplish a specific task.

From a functional point of view public medical care, as defined here, includes all the facilities and services needed by a sick individual, not physicians' services alone. If there is one lesson that can be learned from the rapid advance of medical science and the practical application of scientific knowledge and skill, it is this: the various types of facilities and services necessary to meet adequately the needs of the sick are so closely related to one another and so interdependent, both professionally and economically, that they should be considered as an entity.

Public medical care in the United States has developed from humble beginnings in colonial times to a social movement steadily gaining in impetus. In spite of, and because of, its progress it has been, and continues to be, a controversial issue.

There is little dispute about the principle of public responsibility for adequate medical care. But there are wide differences of opinion as to the extent to which that principle should be applied and the form of organization that would best serve the purposes to be accomplished.

In the course of centuries a large number and bewildering variety of public facilities and services for the sick have evolved. They have grown piecemeal and haphazardly.

At first glance the picture of this development seems to be like a mosaic without any design. Closer study, however, reveals that there are definite patterns. The advance of public medical care has taken place in four principal directions at different rates of speed.

1. A public hospital system, including a large number and great variety of facilities for medical care, has been developed under the auspices of local, state, and Federal governments. It has grown from three main roots: "the pesthouse," the "insane asylum," and the "sick ward" in the workhouse or almshouse.

2. Various types of clinics have evolved out of the primitive dispensary distributing free drugs to the poor.

3. Organized programs, providing for home, office, clinic, hospital, and custodial care at public expense, have been set up for numerous socio-economic groups. They have superseded the old emergency provisions for a tiny segment of the population. In addition, separate programs, including complete medical care, have been established for the control of certain diseases and defects.

4. Responsibility for organization and administration of facilities and services for the care of the sick has been transferred from small to larger political units. Increasing emphasis has been placed on Federal-state and state-local cooperation so as to meet the needs for improvement of public medical care.

In many instances serious efforts have been made to substitute long-term strategy for the stopgap tactics typical of public policy in early times. The attainment of quantitative and qualitative adequacy of public medical care has been realized and accepted as a major task in contrast to the days when governments grudgingly granted a service that was too little, too late, and too poor. Some beginning has been made to bring the public services for the sick into closer relation with the public provisions for the prevention of illness and promotion of good health and to coordinate them with nongovernmental activities. But the development has been fragmentary and far from uniform. Some of the policies and procedures adopted long ago have proved to possess a surprising longevity. They have remained substantially unchanged or have been but slightly modified —in spite of the rapid advance of scientific medicine and the profound social and economic changes that have taken place.

Details on the progress of public policy from the time of the emergence of community responsibility for medical care up to the turning point of the global war will be presented in subsequent chapters.

· 2 ·

THE GROWTH OF PUBLIC HOSPITALS

THE public hospital system in the United States has grown and expanded continuously. In 1942 the registered facilities controlled by local, state, and Federal governments provided 1,015,781 beds, or close to three fourths of all beds available in the country. They rendered service to nearly one third of all hospital admissions and to more than three fourths of the hospital population.[1] These figures are striking and impressive. They furnish conclusive evidence that there is an extensive program of hospital care under public auspices. They do not depict, however, the part played by the public hospital in the community health program. Actually, one in every four governmental hospitals and one in every five beds in them are, as a rule, not available for general use. They are restricted to designated groups of the population for whose care the Federal government has assumed responsibility.

Of the beds in Federal hospitals in 1942, more than three fourths were in general, about one fifth in mental, about one fiftieth in tuberculosis, and an insignificant fraction in other hospitals.

In contrast, about three fourths of the beds maintained by local and state governments were in facilities designated for patients with mental deviations, while about one seventh were in general, about one twelfth in tuberculosis, and a small proportion in various other types of hospitals.

Evidently the course followed by the various public agencies has been quite dissimilar. For selected groups general hospital facilities have been provided in relatively large numbers. For community service, on the other hand, the special hospitals for mental deviations have been the principal facilities established at public expense, while general hospitals have been made available on a relatively very small scale.

The development of hospital facilities under the auspices of local and state agencies has been decisively influenced by the interpretation of government's obligations in this field. Traditionally, provision for selected services—but not the creation of a balanced hospital system—has been considered a public concern.

In early times assumption of community responsibility for institutions was motivated by fear, the need of self-preservation, and the desire to be sparing with expenditures for the maintenance of "paupers." The main objectives of social action were to prevent danger to the community and to salvage human flotsam. In line with this concept facilities were established for the segregation of patients suffering from the diseases most feared, the contagious and mental, and for the accommodation of the destitute sick. They were the first manifestations of public responsibility for institutions. For a long time "the State [closed] its eyes to all illnesses which did not fit the crude conception which identified the sick person with the criminal and removed him for the while from society, not for his reformation, but for the public good." [2] This comment, made by J. H. Harley Williams on the social philosophy prevailing in Great Britain up to the turn of the nineteenth century, can be applied to many a country.

The old public institutions were designed and equipped to give custodial care only, and that at a minimum expense to the taxpayer. Shocking defects in building, equipment, and care were frequent; time and again they aroused public indignation. But the niggardly attitude of official agencies toward their institutions for the sick prevented radical improvements. The reasons for this attitude were anything but obscure. The diseases recognized as requiring institutionalization at public expense were those which were believed to demand nothing but custodial care. The carefully restricted group of the sick admitted, the destitute, were regarded as an inevitable burden to the taxpayer and were provided only with the minimum of care.

No respectable citizen would descend to such depths as to apply for admission to a public institution if he could help it.

In the course of the nineteenth century, particularly towards the end, the picture began to change. Scientific and technical progress made it possible to transform the old institution for the sick from a center of danger into a center of usefulness. Four developments combined to make the modern hospital. They were: improvement of sanitary conditions; progress in architectural design and construction; advance in diagnosis, treatment, and medical technique; and introduction of organized professional services by physicians, nurses, and medical social workers. It must be noted that "medical social service in hospitals" in the modern sense is a product of the twentieth century.

The functions of a hospital could be redefined. Around the middle of the nineteenth century the institution for bed patients was still generally believed to serve three major purposes. Rudolf Virchow described them as follows: to furnish custodial care for the sick; to provide for the professional education of medical and nursing students; and to carry out medical research. A generation later it had become clear that the modern hospital could make another, and highly important, contribution to society as well as to the individual: namely, organizing and providing adequate and competent diagnostic and treatment service. Restoration of health, working ability, and earning capacity became a new and increasingly stressed objective of hospitalization.

The contemporary concept of a hospital is well expressed in the following definition:

[A hospital is] a community organization which provides facilities and personnel for rendering the highest possible grade of health services to patients, professional groups and the community; for educating the community to demand and support adequate health services and sound health policies, for educating additional personnel and professional groups in technical fields and in co-operative endeavor; and for advancing our knowledge of disease and its prevention through technical research and appropriate organization.[3]

Huge was the task faced by communities anxious to keep pace with scientific and technological progress. There were new opportunities to improve the situation in the hospital field. But there arose also a big problem. Should tax funds be raised and allotted only to reorganize, modernize, and increase such services as were traditionally supported by local and state governments or should a broader policy be adopted? The decision fell in favor of a new approach. Since the end of the nineteenth century public policy in regard to hospitals has changed markedly.

Communities became cognizant of needs hitherto disregarded. Many abandoned the time-honored concept that the establishment of facilities for communicable diseases and mental deviations and the provision of free service for the poor were the standard and only functions of government in the field of hospitalization. More diseases and special conditions were added to the list of those warranting hospital care at public expense. Among them, physical handicaps and malignant tumors received primary consideration. Determined efforts were made to substitute general hospitals meeting modern standards for institutions of the poorhouse type.

New principles of organizing facilities for the care of the sick emerged. In the first place, differentiation of service according to special needs was emphasized. A variety of special hospitals were established and gradually subdivided into units designated and equipped to perform particular functions. General hospitals were departmentalized, often to a high degree. Unfortunately, the principle of specialized service has not been carried far enough. Chronic disease and convalescent hospitals have been sadly neglected. Secondly, concentration of highly specialized personnel, equipment, and physical plants was stressed in the interest of optimum and economical utilization of all resources. Hospitals of moderate or large size have been built in preference to small ones that cannot be equipped and staffed adequately and still be operated economically.

In general, the special hospitals under government control, such as tuberculosis and mental hospitals, have been staffed with salaried physicians. On the other hand, most of the general hospitals have only a skeleton staff of full-time physicians and rely for professional services largely on physicians practicing in the community.

In short, the public hospital system, once comprising a few types of special facilities, began to expand along all fronts. What is even more significant, many of the governmental hospitals reached a high standard, chiefly as a result of harmonious cooperation between public agencies and the American College of Surgeons. Others, however, continued to be ugly ducklings among local facilities.

Increasingly the services of hospitals controlled by local and state governments were made available to the public at large rather than merely to the needy. Such opportunity was first offered to patients with communicable or mental diseases and gradually, although not uniformly, extended to others regardless of the type of disease. The long-standing distinction between these special hospitals for all of the people and general hospitals for the poor became less sharp; in some parts of the country it has disappeared. Particularly in small towns and sparsely populated areas has the governmental hospital become a true community hospital providing medical care for all economic groups.

In hundreds of communities a service once disliked, if not despised, by all has won a high place in public esteem and is used by people from all walks of life. Yet, there are instances where governmental facilities demonstrated an old truth to be valid: evil reputations cannot be lost in decades, while good reputations can be lost over night. In some large cities the municipal general hospital, deservedly or not, has remained separated from the community by a wall of distrust.

A similar change took place in Great Britain, once called "the home of the voluntary hospital." [4] Prior to 1929, only infectious disease, mental, and poor-law hospitals were supported out of tax funds. Since the early thirties public general hospitals for community use have been provided on the basis of a carefully drawn plan. They have grown in number, improved in quality, and won the confidence of the people.

FACILITIES FOR PATIENTS WITH COMMUNICABLE DISEASES

Community responsibility for establishment of institutional facilities for communicable diseases dates far back. It has advanced particularly since the Middle Ages when severe epidemics struck many European countries and created problems of tremendous gravity and magnitude. *Visis effectibus*, after the effect of epidemics had been seen, communities tried to prevent the recurrence of devastating visitations from a disease that *communicat multitudini*. The two principal methods employed were maritime quarantine, that is, the detention for a fixed period of all vessels coming from an infected port, and isolation of the infectious sick in special institutions established for this purpose.

American policy followed the same path. Public responsibility for maintenance of isolation facilities was increasingly accepted in the eighteenth century. Stirred by the staggering toll in human lives and the havoc wrought to business by "contagious" diseases, public opinion strongly demanded and unreservedly endorsed the allocation of tax funds so as to eliminate the danger to public health. One community after another adopted statutes authorizing or requiring the maintenance of special institutions, such as pesthouses, lazarettos, or smallpox hospitals. These institutions became the favorite places for exiling the sick from the rest of the community. They were complemented by facilities at seaports for the detention of passengers and crews suspected of "a contagious distemper," as the quarantine law enacted by the colonial legislature of New York in 1758 put it. Objectives other than these were temporarily attained with the introduction of inoculation hospitals designed to provide for inoculation against smallpox.

Definite as the interest in community responsibility was, it occurred in waves, gaining momentum with a new outbreak and slowing down with the disappearance of an epidemic. Action was taken only if and when an emergency arose. Temporary arrangements and makeshift solutions were the rule. Facilities were maintained "for the duration" and discontinued when the scare subsided. Simple expedients were employed, such as the conversion of refuges, almshouses, inns, or doctors' homes into temporary isolation facilities or the use of hastily erected barracks or camps. As late as 1897, Kern County in California saw only one way out of the dilemma created by a smallpox epidemic: to isolate the patients in tents out on the plains and have them watched by an armed guard to prevent their escape.[5]

Isolation facilities were mainly for patients who were recognized as affected with a highly communicable disease. Wards in workhouses or poorhouses accommodated many destitute patients in an infectious stage whose condition was not noticed at all or believed to warrant no special attention. In the absence of any provision for isolation these "fever cases" made the institutions into centers from which infection spread. Most of the hospitals, primarily those of the proprietary and nonprofit voluntary type, for reasons of self-protection refused to admit any patients with an infectious disease or transferred them immediately after the diagnosis was established. Significantly, in the French capital in 1893, the general hospitals La Pitié with 766 beds and La Charité with 520 beds had but five and three isolation rooms respectively. The dangerous conditions prevailing in the hospitals of many countries by the end of the nineteenth century were summed up by M. L. Davis at the International Congress of Charities, Correction, and Philanthropy held in Chicago in 1893 in the following words: "The labors of sanitarians have been directed almost exclusively towards preventing the spread of disease from the sick to the well—no attempt being made to protect those already ill from receiving more of the disease germs and, thereby, aggravating each individual case."[6]

A new phase of development began late in the nineteenth century. Permanent programs emphasizing adequate and competent treatment to render infectious patients noninfectious superseded temporary arrangements for the segregation of such patients as were highly contagious. The scientific basis for the turn to new objectives was provided by the rapid progress in the knowledge of causation and modes of transmission of infection; the adoption of new principles of hospital building; the vast improvement in the technique of care of infectious patients; and, last but not least, the introduction of new and effective treatment methods. All these advances made it possible to build up an entirely different system of hospital care.

The old isolation facilities had served "contagious" patients without distinction as to type of disease, although there had been some exceptions to the rule. Particularly notable are the special institutions for syphilitic patients maintained by a number of cities on the European continent as early as the end of the fifteenth century and the smallpox hospitals established later in many countries.

The new policy was based on the principle of organizing special services to meet the special needs resulting from specific diseases.

Four main types of facilities for patients with communicable diseases have come into use: (1) special hospitals designed exclusively for the treatment and care of a large variety of acute infectious diseases; (2) special hospitals accepting exclusively patients with a distinct type of infection such as tuberculosis or venereal disease; (3) general hospitals and special facilities, such as mental or children's hospitals, equipped with units for service to a variety of infectious patients; and (4) special institutions designed primarily for long isolation of patients with conditions such as leprosy or advanced tuberculosis in a chronic stage.

These facilities are distinguished by their functions as well as by the type of disease admitted. The first three groups emphasize treatment, including that of complicated conditions, and, to a varying extent, observation for the establishment of diagnosis. Isolation remains, of course, an important objective. The fourth group places the main emphasis on segregation so as to prevent danger to the community but also makes provisions for medical supervision and such treatment as may be needed. It includes a variety of institutions ranging from simple homelike facilities to elaborate settlement-like organizations.

In organizing treatment services for patients with communicable diseases other than tuberculosis (and, sometimes, venereal disease) the various countries have applied fundamentally different principles.

Great Britain, along with a group of other countries, such as Sweden, decided to concentrate all patients with acute infectious diseases in special "infectious disease hospitals." Many of them were developed by reorganization of the old "pesthouses" and "fever hospitals." Isolation wards in general hospitals and special institutions were maintained only to a relatively limited extent. Their bed capacity was kept at the level sufficient to permit observation of patients with suspected infection and meet the contingency of infectious cases arising among the patients admitted until transfer could be effectuated. In 1936 there were about 1,000 infectious disease hospitals with about 40,000 beds, and these included over 300 smallpox hospitals with nearly 7,000 beds.[7] All were controlled by public authorities. Significantly, about seventy years earlier most of the "fever hospitals" had been maintained by nongovernmental organizations.

Scrutinizing the various approaches to "the most perfect hospital program" for communicable diseases, the United States and a group of other countries have come to emphasize a policy sharply contrasting with that exemplified by the British. In 1927 (the first year for which accurate information is available) only 98 isolation hospitals with 8,895 beds were listed on the register of the American Medical Association. By 1942 their number had declined to 52 and their bed capacity to 6,279. These beds represented less than one half of one per cent of all beds in registered hospitals and about 0.6 per cent of all those in public hospitals. Some communities maintained small separate isolation facilities not included in the register. All but two of the registered isolation hospitals were supported by public agencies; about three fourths of those under public control were owned by cities, most of the rest by counties, and a few were under city-county control.

Admitted to isolation hospitals are all or most of the communicable diseases, as defined by the United States Public Health Service,[8] although in some instances either tuberculosis or venereal diseases or both are excluded. The following are examples of different admission policies:

The Philadelphia Hospital for Contagious Diseases in Philadelphia, Pennsylvania, a city institution of more than 900 beds, admits all communicable diseases except venereal diseases. "Incorrigible tuberculosis patients" are committed by the Municipal Court on charges brought against them by the Department of Health.

The Essex County Hospital for Contagious Diseases in Belleville, New Jersey, a county institution of about 500 beds, admits all communicable diseases, including acute gonorrhea, syphilis in the primary and secondary stages, and tuberculosis in children up to the age of fourteen.

The Oakland County Contagious Hospital in Pontiac, Michigan, a county institution of 85 beds, admits all communicable diseases including venereal diseases but excluding tuberculosis.

What types of disease are the leading causes of admission depends on many factors. Of prime importance are the prevalence of certain diseases and the occurrence of epidemics in a particular area; the common concepts on the relative value of hospitalization or home care of certain diseases; and the policies as to payment for needed service.

The Philadelphia Hospital for Contagious Diseases, in the years 1940 to 1942, reported scarlet fever as the leading cause of admission, accounting for about two thirds to three fourths of all. The Essex County Hospital for Contagious Diseases listed measles and scarlet fever as the diseases most frequently admitted in the years 1940 and 1941. These diseases together constituted approximately half of all admissions. In the Oakland County Contagious Hospital in 1942 patients with scarlet fever made up by far the largest single group and those with genital gonorrhea the second largest group admitted.

In 1942, the reported admissions to registered isolation hospitals in the United States were 37,936 as against 40,210 in 1931, the first year for which more reliable figures were recorded. They accounted for about 0.3 per cent of all hospital admissions. There was ample space in the isolation hospitals, though. On the average, only about 40 per cent of the available bed capacity was occupied—a proportion rarely exceeded during the preceding ten years. On the other hand, about 2,823,000 cases of communicable diseases, including about 119,000 cases of tuberculosis and about 785,000 cases of gonorrhea and syphilis, were reported in 1942 in the United States. Where hospital care was indicated it was provided. But it was the general hospital rather than the isolation hospital that was primarily used to hospitalize the patient.

During the last decades increasing emphasis has been placed on the development of adequate facilities for the care of infectious patients in close functional and administrative connection with general and special hospitals of various types. Separate units on the same grounds with or in proximity to the main hospital or separate wings and wards or single rooms located in the main building have been provided in large numbers. The "special features required for the communicable disease unit" of a general hospital have been outlined by the Committee on Hospital Planning and Equipment of the American Hospital Association.[9]

Such a method of organization, if properly applied, is believed to offer great advantages, both scientific and economic. It makes the services of specialists from other departments readily available for diagnosis and treatment; renders it unnecessary to transport patients long distances and to transfer them from one hospital to another in case of complications; allows for flexibility in utilizing beds according to actual needs; avoids stigmatization of hospital and patients; and may serve to reduce the costs of operating and administering the unit. However, if several hospitals in the same area provide such service, they ought to agree on a joint plan for admission of patients with communicable diseases, each hospital concentrating on certain types. Else much of the benefit that can be derived from specialization would be lost.

In line with this change in concepts general and special hospitals, primarily those under government control, were reorganized and equipped to perform effectively the function of serving patients with communicable diseases. What is even more significant, a noteworthy rapprochement between official agencies and other groups active in the hospital field took place. In a considerable number of instances public authorities aided voluntary hospitals by land donations, subsidies from tax funds or both in constructing, enlarging, or improving facilities for patients with communicable diseases. In other instances they built, at public expense, a special unit on the grounds of the voluntary institution but left its operation and use to the hospital on the condition that a certain number of beds would be reserved for free service to the needy.

The result of all these efforts is that in the United States at present the special units in general and special hospitals and in various institutions together contribute by far the largest share to the services for patients with communicable diseases except tuberculosis. They furnish more than 39,000 beds, nine tenths of which are in governmental hospitals.

To serve the community health program effectively, a public hospital with facilities for the care of patients with communicable diseases must admit everybody, regardless of income and place of residence.

In isolated instances communities have early shown a remarkably progressive attitude in defining the conditions under which public facilities could be used by persons suffering from a "contagious" disease. In 1496, the German city of Nuremberg, later degraded to a shrine of Nazism, converted a refuge for migrants and destitute persons into a special institution for the treatment of patients with *Malafranzos*, that is, syphilis. Paying patients as well as the poor and nonresidents as well as residents were accepted. The nonresidents, however, were discharged from the institution and expelled from the city as soon as they were able to walk; they were forbidden to re-enter city territory until they were well.[10]

In Great Britain it was not until 1879 that the Poor Law Act was amended to allow the admission of "nonpaupers" to a "fever hospital." The need for such a revision of the official policy had been amply demonstrated by the experience during the great smallpox epidemic of 1870–71. Nine tenths of the persons admitted to the institutions of the Metropolitan Asylum Board were found to have become paupers only for the sake of gaining entrance.

The situation prevailing in the United States at the end of the nineteenth century was discussed by G. H. M. Rowe before the International Congress of Charities, Correction, and Philanthropy held in Chicago in 1893. Rowe referred to a question raised in a popular magazine: "Where is the place to which a lady living in a boarding house or temporarily stopping at a hotel could take her child affected with scarlet fever?" All he could answer was this: "To the best of my knowledge, Boston is the only large city where a hotel guest or a citizen in good circumstances can obtain suitable accommodation in a hospital, if he is ill with diphtheria, scarlet fever or small-pox. In most cities the better class of corporate general hospitals absolutely refuse him admission." [11]

Since the turn of the century the rules governing admission to a governmental facility for communicable diseases have been generally changed. Jurisdictional and economic considerations have been ranked second to the objective of controlling infection. The distinction between residents and nonresidents has been abandoned in principle, although there are differences in practice. Some hospitals are restricted to people residing in a county, others to those living within a state. However, no limitations apply if an individual from some distant location requires immediate hospital care. As a general rule, patients are accepted regardless of their economic condition. Those able to pay are charged the rates fixed by the hospital, and those unable to contribute to the costs of their care receive service at public expense. In determining eligibility for free care liberal practices are the rule if hospitalization is necessary to protect the public from danger. Such interpretation allows for considerable latitude of action on the part of public agencies. On the other hand, stiff eligibility requirements may be applied if the case of a patient is construed differently. The statutes in effect in Minnesota afford a vivid illustration of the difficulties created by administrative distinction between measures for the common good and service for the welfare of the individual.

The Minnesota law sets forth that the cost of protecting the public from communicable diseases, including the cost of hospitalization for this purpose, is a proper charge (when the patient himself cannot pay) upon the town, village, or city, which may in turn recover from the county one half of the amount paid. Measures employed for the care, comfort, or relief of the patient, but not necessary for the protection of the public, must be paid by the patient or from relief funds.

If it is true that the widest possible use of hospital care is one of the prerequisites to the prevention of the spread of communicable diseases, then one conclusion is inescapable: hospitalization for communicable diseases ought to be available either free or at low rates for everybody; at least it ought to be provided for the common man and without forcing him to apply for relief. Such policies have been adopted in a score of foreign countries. Community responsibility is assumed not only for the establishment of facilities but also for the payment of the greater part of their operating costs, and the national government contributes to the cost of both building and maintenance. In Sweden, for example, in 1940 tax funds defrayed all but about one and one-half per cent of the expenditures for operating 138 communicable disease hospitals with 6,295 beds.

FACILITIES FOR PATIENTS WITH TUBERCULOSIS

The founding of the first institution designed exclusively for the treatment of tuberculosis of the lungs antedated the discovery of the tubercle bacillus by several decades. In England, Dr. George Bodington, as early as 1840, presented the idea of special facilities for tuberculous patients and emphasized the importance of out-of-door life. His efforts to develop a sanatorium failed. It was a German physician who succeeded in molding public opinion. In 1854, Hermann Brehmer, a young doctor suffering from tuberculosis, settled in Görbersdorf, Silesia, to prove the theory expounded in his doctoral dissertation: "phthisis is curable." [12] Three years later he was able to report that pulmonary tuberculosis could be cured under certain conditions. What was necessary for this purpose was a special facility exclusively for tuberculosis patients.[13] Brehmer opened his own sanatorium in 1858, and a few other farseeing men followed suit. Salubrious climate, fresh air, sunshine, diet, graduated exercise in the open air, and carefully scheduled bed rest (introduced by Peter Dettweiler), all applied strictly according to the condition of the individual and supervised by the physician—these were the means by which the pioneers hoped to accomplish the desired end.

History repeated itself in the United States when another young physician, Edward L. Trudeau, also a victim of tuberculosis, independently succeeded in arresting his own disease by the same method as that employed by Brehmer and his disciples. In 1882 he read of his German colleagues' ideas and practices and decided to follow them. Three years later he was able to open the first tuberculosis sanatorium in the United States, originally known as the Adirondack Cottage Sanitarium, at Saranac Lake in New York State.[14]

The basic principle of sanatorium treatment extolled by the pioneers stood the test of time, even though later better knowledge of the various factors involved resulted in their revaluation and a more accurate appraisal of their relative merits. Sanatoria were established in increasing numbers and soon came to occupy a dominant place in the institutional program for tuberculous patients. To direct the movement into proper channels, the American Sanatorium Association and the National Tuberculosis Association in 1927 issued a set of minimum standards for tuberculosis sanatoria, designed for self-rating by the hospital.

Gradually more types of specialized treatment facilities were developed. Particularly noticeable was the introduction of specially organized, staffed, and equipped tuberculosis units at general hospitals and, also, at mental, isolation, and other special hospitals. In 1938, according to the first nearly complete survey, there were 1,140 tuberculosis facilities in the United States. About 42 per cent were sanatoria, about 55 per cent hospital departments, and the remainder preventoria. The available beds totalled 98,801 and included 87,084 for adults and 11,717 for children. Close to three fourths were in sanatoria; of those in tuberculosis departments the majority were in general hospitals.[15]

Marked as the progress was in general, it was far from uniform. The distribution of tuberculosis facilities had remained very uneven. Beds were relatively numerous in wealthy parts and rare in poor sections of the country—the very areas where the need was greatest as manifested by the incidence and mortality from the disease. In 1939 beds in tuberculosis hospitals, excluding facilities in general hospitals, were available at the rate of 0.59 per 1,000 of the population or 1.27 for every tuberculosis death reported.[16] The standards of the Committee on Administrative Practice of the American Public Health Association call for an average of two beds per annual death. This requirement, also stressed in *The Need for a National Health Program*,[17] was met in only eleven states while six states had less than half a bed per death.

With the development of a variety of institutional services for tuberculous patients, definition and demarcation of their functions became a necessity. As experience with the results of sanatorium treatment accumulated, the potentialities of this type of care could be gauged. As scientific knowledge of prevention, diagnosis, treatment, and care of tuberculosis advanced, it became possible to determine the part to be played by each of the treatment facilities in the total program of tuberculosis control.

The functions of the tuberculosis hospital, as they have evolved in the United States up to the early thirties, have been described by Philip P. Jacobs as follows: prevention of infection; education of the patient; cure or arrest of tuberculosis; training of doctors and nurses; economic rehabilitation of the patient; humane care of the sick who cannot be restored to their homes; diagnostic center; prevention of tuberculosis in children; and medical and social research in tuberculosis.[18] Here, only the development of treatment services will be briefly reviewed.

In the first phase of the sanatorium movement all stages of tuberculosis were admitted; inevitably advanced cases exceeded in number all others. Isolation and humane care of the seriously ill were objectives strongly emphasized, although administration of the unspecific treatment regime, as outlined by the pioneers, was not neglected. Official agencies expected the sick to stay until they were no longer "dangerous to the public health." Gradually a tendency developed to give primary consideration to patients offering a reasonable prospect of recovery, particularly those in an early stage, and to limit the proportion of advanced cases.

An entirely new phase was ushered in with the introduction of surgical methods, primarily of collapse therapy, into the treatment scheme of tuberculosis of the lungs. Moderately advanced and, to some extent, even far advanced cases now could be treated successfully and, therefore, be accepted with less reluctance. The proportion of "hopeless cases" was steadily decreasing.

The development of surgical treatment could not fail to exert a profound influence on the method of building sanatoria. Not only were permanent constructions substituted for the original makeshift accommodations but many sanatoria grew to become essentially hospitals, equipped for all types of service. Increasingly, new tuberculosis facilities were laid out, constructed, organized, and operated like general hospitals. To avoid waste of effort and attain optimum efficiency in the use of highly specialized personnel and facilities, emphasis was placed upon the establishment of plants of moderate rather than small size.

Where the sanatorium continued to limit the scope of its services, the tuberculosis department in general hospitals took responsibility for complementary work. It provided for observation of doubtful cases, preparation of patients for sanatorium cure, operative work, and care of the sick in a terminal stage.

These advances in the organization of institutional services did not solve one problem that was uppermost in the minds of many experts. "What is needed is not more isolation but isolation of more persons"—this doctrine, it was widely believed, ought to be applied to tuberculosis by utilizing the special hospitals for extensive and protracted segregation of infectious patients.

THE GROWTH OF PUBLIC HOSPITALS

Robert Koch, in his last paper written shortly before his death, pointed out that the tremendous number of tuberculous adults constituted a serious obstacle to the hospitalization of even a large fraction of such patients.[19] Later experience brought some more aspects of the problem to light. The costs of establishing and operating tuberculosis facilities meeting modern standards had been mounting by necessity. Was it inevitable that the building program should be expanded so as to overcome the chronic shortage of beds? Was it economical to use highly specialized and costly services for the isolation of chronic infectious patients over a long period of time only to aggravate the scarcity of beds so badly needed for active treatment? Was hospitalization in itself the appropriate method for meeting the needs of patients lacking decent and healthful living accommodations, adequate diet, nursing care, regular medical supervision, and an opportunity to utilize their limited capacity to work? Should and could hospitals apply force to detain patients acting in such an irresponsible manner as to endanger their families and the community?

So formidable appeared the practical difficulties to be overcome in answering these questions that action was slow to be taken. In a few countries a beginning in a new direction has been made. Separate homelike facilities for the care of patients in an advanced stage have been provided sporadically, particularly in Norway [20] and Denmark. Village settlements, including work colonies, have been established as part of the tuberculosis hospital in a few countries. The English colonies have attracted particular attention.[21]

Countries harassed by the "white plague" should have been expected to be quick in organizing their institutional services for tuberculosis of the lungs by concerted action of all groups concerned. Yet, until the end of the nineteenth century this overwhelming task was generally left to the efforts of voluntary organizations. In some countries the disregard of the tuberculous patient's special needs as well as of the community's welfare was in marked contrast to the scientific contributions that were made. Italy, whose Carlo Forlanini had won wide fame for promoting the application of artificial pneumothorax since 1882, possessed, two years later, only one hospital for tuberculous patients—and that was closed for repair. At the same time most of her general hospitals refused admission to such patients. Germany, the country where Robert Koch discovered the tubercle bacillus in 1882 and Wilhelm Roentgen the X rays in 1895, long relied on the leadership of voluntary agencies and the semipublic, autonomous organizations administering social insurance with the result that community-wide programs did not evolve.

In the twentieth century a new social philosophy came to the fore. Governmental agencies increasingly appropriated funds for the erection of tuberculosis wards at general or other hospitals and for the building of separate tuberculosis facilities. The efforts were concentrated on the development of special hospitals, on the theory they were "the battleground of the war against tuberculosis" and the hub of all treatment services. Within a relatively short period of time public responsibility superseded private responsibility for provision of institutional services.

In Great Britain in 1937 close to three fourths of all tuberculosis beds in sanatoria, isolation hospitals, general hospitals, and poor-law institutions were in facilities controlled by public agencies. In the United States in 1938 about 83 per cent of all beds in sanatoria, hospital departments, and preventoria were in institutions owned by governmental agencies. The large majority of the governmental sanatoria had 100 beds or more, while about one seventh had fewer than 50 beds. On the other hand, many of the tuberculosis departments in governmental hospitals had less than 25 beds.

The admission policy to tuberculosis hospitals under government control is not uniform throughout the United States. In some states the public facilities are available without regard to the financial condition of the patient; in others they are restricted to persons who cannot pay for care in private institutions and in still others to "indigent" patients. Nevertheless, the determination of eligibility is made in a liberal way.

Where there are no economic restrictions on admission, patients with resources of their own are required to pay the full charges or such portion as they can. In general, the rates are set relatively low in order to prevent the family from breaking down under the weight of high expenditures for long drawn out treatment. Persons who themselves or through relatives cannot pay any part of the costs charged receive care at public expense. As the number of free beds in some hospitals is limited, poor patients not infrequently have to wait for months until they can be accepted.

The principle of community responsibility for the payment of service furnished either by a governmental or a nongovernmental hospital has received undisputed public support. In 1935 tax funds accounted for 77.8 per cent of the income of all registered tuberculosis hospitals (excluding those under Federal control), while patients contributed 14.3 per cent and other sources 7.9 per cent. It is noteworthy that the nongovernmental tuberculosis hospitals received approximately one fourth of their income from taxes.[22]

Small communities usually do not need many tuberculosis beds nor are they able to support a tuberculosis hospital worthy of the name. This fact has been generally recognized. All civilized countries have taken steps to spread the financial burden of establishing high-grade tuberculosis facilities. The broad policies adopted reveal two patterns.

In the first place, larger political units or geographic areas were authorized or required to provide for tuberculosis hospitals at public expense. In Sweden, for instance, responsibility was vested in the provincial councils. In the United States in 1942 primarily states and counties and to a lesser extent cities and city-county organizations operated such facilities for community use; the Federal government owned specialized services for designated beneficiaries. Forty-two states maintained their own tuberculosis hospitals as compared with one in 1895. Massachusetts had been the pioneer. The state institutions contained the relatively largest number and proportion of beds provided under public auspices, closely followed by county institutions.

But even larger communities and commonwealths, if their per capita income is low, find it difficult to raise the funds required for provision of up-to-date tuberculosis hospitals. Failure to adjust public policy to new requirements has greatly retarded the general progress of institutional services for tuberculosis in many countries. In a number of instances, however, the traditional concepts on distribution of responsibility among various levels of government have been revised. The obligation of the national government to aid in the construction and equipment of adequate tuberculosis facilities has been acknowledged in a score of foreign countries. This constitutes the second trend of basic importance.

Norway, Denmark, and Sweden, in 1900, 1905, and 1908 respectively, adopted the principle that the national government had to share in the costs of sanatoria built and operated by local agencies.

Other European countries, Belgium, France, and Switzerland, have followed suit since the second decade of this century. Great Britain began in 1912 to make annual grants-in-aid from national funds to local authorities for a variety of activities in connection with tuberculosis control, including the provision of additional beds in special institutions. By an act of 1921 the local authorities were charged with the duty of providing treatment service for all tuberculous patients on a community-wide basis. The passage of the Local Government Act in 1929, the most important landmark in the development of public medical care in Great Britain, brought with it a considerable extension of financial aid for provision, extension, and modernization of tuberculosis institutions of various types.

FACILITIES FOR PATIENTS WITH MENTAL DEVIATIONS

For a long time provision of adequate institutional care for the mentally sick and defective has received little attention. Even in advanced countries it is still far from satisfactory.

Four conspicuous developments mark the line of progress. Highly specialized facilities have been developed for several types of mental deviation. Institutions for the mentally sick have been transformed into hospitals in fact as well as in name. Public responsibility has been accepted for the establishment of necessary facilities and the regulation of nongovernmental activities in this field. The services of governmental hospitals have been made available to everybody regardless of economic considerations.

The advance, greatly varying in rate and speed, has been one of kind rather than of degree. The attitude toward mental deviations in general and their institutional care in particular is indicated by the official language employed at various periods. In the early days it was common in the English speaking countries to use the terms "lunatic asylum" and "insane hospital." The oldest American hospital for the mentally sick was authorized by an act of the Virginia House of Burgesses in 1770 to "make provision for the support and maintenance of idiots, lunatics, and other persons of unsound minds." It opened in 1773 as "The Public Hospital for Persons of Insane and Disordered Mind," changed its name in 1841 to "Eastern Lunatic Asylum," and finally, in 1894, was renamed "Eastern State Hospital."

Newer scientific concepts penetrated the cloud banks of tradition with extreme slowness. In the United States, statutes and administrative rules, with a few notable exceptions, still refer to "lunacy" or "insanity," and such time-honored expressions as "keeper" for attendant and "inmate discharged on parole" for tentatively discharged patient are widely used. In England the old terminology was discarded in 1930 when the "mental patient" and the "mental hospital" were officially introduced into modern society.

Old records reveal another concept that exerted a profound and lasting influence on the attitude of official agencies toward persons with mental deviations. In 1641 American pioneers inserted in "The Body of Liberties of the Colony of Massachusetts Bay" the following item: "children, idiots, distracted persons, and all that are strangers, or new comers to our plantation, shall have such allowances and dispensations in any cause whether criminal or other as religion and reason require." [23] The classification of the mentally sick and defective together with other persons presumed to require aid was quite in line with the knowledge and practices of the time. The same idea still shaped public policy in the second half of the nineteenth century. It was quite common to conduct the almshouse as an asylum for the harmless and incurable insane, the crippled, the epileptic, idiotic children, and for such other persons who on account of their infirmities were unable to support themselves.

Only slowly was it realized that mental deviation was neither a sin nor a crime nor a disgrace, but a disease requiring special service; that hospital care had to be provided for persons other than those with gross mental deviations lest the fight be waged badly; and that disease rather than poverty was the reasonable starting point for community action.

In the United States, as in many other countries, the principle of differentiating services according to special needs was applied to patients with mental deviations sporadically late in the eighteenth century, infrequently in the first half of the nineteenth century, and on a larger scale only since the end of the nineteenth century. Before the movement gained momentum practices originating in colonial times had dominated the scene.[24]

In the absence of other facilities the police station had been widely used to "receive" mental patients, and the jail had become the favorite place for the incarceration of those who were dangerous. An ingenious device was employed by some communities on the West

Coast. Around 1850 San Francisco and Stockton "accommodated" their mental patients aboard abandoned vessels lying in harbor until a place in a jail or "hospital" became free.[25] Even today the jail often serves as waiting room for the mentally sick pending their transportation to a hospital.

Workhouses, too, had been utilized extensively. To give an example, in 1727 a Connecticut act stipulated that individuals "under distraction and unfit to go at large" be confined in the colony workhouse. In a later phase the almshouse came to occupy a prominent place in the institutional program supported by tax funds. Mentally sick and defective persons without resources of their own were huddled together with other poor persons, and the violent were confined in strait jackets. An appalling mass of human wreckage congregated in these places. Telling are the figures given for Michigan. "It was estimated, in 1873, that of an average poorhouse population of fifteen hundred persons, two hundred and fifty were insane, one hundred and twenty-five were idiots, forty were blind, twenty were mute, and about three hundred were epileptic or had deformities or chronic diseases."[26] When, in 1915, the Connecticut legislature passed an act requiring towns to "have all inmates of almshouses examined twice a year to discover any insane or feeble-minded," a problem was touched which had not been confined to that state. In fact, as late as 1940, many mental defectives could be found in orphanages, almshouses, and homes for the aged—not to mention correctional institutions—and quite a few mentally sick in places such as nursing homes and poorhouses.

The first hospitals designed exclusively for the care of the sick also were unspecialized. The Pennsylvania Hospital in Philadelphia, opened in 1752, had the ground floor reserved for mental patients and the two upper floors for others. The governors of the New York Hospital, for which the cornerstone was laid in 1773, provided in 1774 "that the Comm. for Superintending the Building be Authorized to Appropriate the Cellar part of the North Building . . . into wards or Cells, for the reception of Lunatics."[27] Special provisions for the mentally sick were made in 1808; a separate building was erected which later developed into the Bloomingdale Hospital, now at White Plains.

Up to the end of the eighteenth century American policy followed the pattern set in European countries. Two typical examples will serve to show how the problem of institutional care for the mentally sick had been approached there. The French Hôtel Dieu, in the fourteenth century, admitted maternity cases, foundlings, old people, and the mentally sick; later it accepted also prostitutes with venereal disease. The Spital zu St. Marx in Vienna performed similar functions up to the turn of the eighteenth century.

The contemporary institutional program for persons with mental deviations includes two basically different categories of facilities: one group designed for patients with mental illness and a second for persons with defective intelligence, particularly children. The facilities for the mentally sick are of four types. They are: (1) the special hospital, organized in separate units with patients' buildings grouped in various styles, and equipped to perform specific functions for various types and stages of illness; (2) the hospital admitting exclusively patients with a special type of illness such as neurosis, epilepsy, or alcohol or drug addiction; (3) wards or departments in general hospitals primarily used for observation, diagnosis, and treatment over a limited period of time; (4) divisions in correctional institutions.

The extent to which specialized services have been developed is remarkable. So is the relatively short period of time that was needed to overcome the growing pains. Sixty-six special facilities for mental disease were in operation in the United States by 1870. In 1942, nervous and mental hospitals registered by the American Medical Association numbered 586.

Marked as the increase in the number of special hospitals was, it was far surpassed by the growth in bed capacity. In 1942, beds reported in registered mental and nervous hospitals numbered 646,118 as against 373,364 beds in 1927, the first year for which more accurate information was compiled. Numerically they exceeded all other groups of hospitalization facilities. Proportionately they accounted for nearly half of all hospital beds: 46.7 per cent in 1942 as against 43.7 per cent in 1927. The special facilities not only have become more numerous, they have grown larger and larger. Considerably more than four fifths of the beds were in facilities with over 1,000 beds, while only less than one per cent were in the relatively numerous institutions with fewer than 50 beds. The beds available in registered and nonregistered mental and nervous hospitals in 1939 averaged 4.59 per 1,000 of the population. Their distribution was very uneven. There were extremes such as 1.79 beds per 1,000 population in one state and 7.47 in another. Only fourteen states had a bed rate of 5.50 or more. The standard recommended by the Committee on the Costs of Medical Care and again emphasized in *The Need for a National Health Program* calls for an average of about 5.6 beds per 1,000 persons.

More recently, mainly since 1920, psychiatric services also have been organized in general hospitals. At the end of 1941, about 5,700 patients with mental diseases were reported to be under treatment in 87 general hospitals. They accounted for about 14 per cent of the average daily population of the reporting institutions.[28]

Public authorities have played a decisive role in these developments after a long period in which they had tried to evade responsibility. They subsidized the building of nongovernmental facilities; took over hospitals founded by pioneering private groups; and established institutions of their own. Around 1870, of the 66 mental hospitals in operation in the United States, 50 with a bed capacity estimated at 13,000 to 14,000 were under government control. In 1939, 96.6 per cent of the beds in mental and nervous hospitals (registered and nonregistered) were in governmental hospitals. These facilities constituted less than 60 per cent of all mental hospitals. Institutional provision for persons with mental deviations thus has become a monopoly of government. The public institutions usually are very large. They are concentrated in the more thickly settled areas and provide more than twice as many beds per unit of population in the wealthy states as in states with low per capita income. The advance in this field has been responsible for much of the increase in the total bed capacity provided at the expense of the taxpayer. In 1942, nearly 62 per cent of all beds in public facilities were in mental and nervous hospitals. In addition, the majority of psychiatric services in general hospitals were under government control.

In Great Britain the development has taken a similar course. Before the war governmental hospitals furnished nearly all of the beds for the mentally sick and defective. In New Zealand all but one small mental hospital are owned by the government.

The policy of substituting specialized for unspecialized facilities was accompanied by efforts to revise the methods of building, equipping, staffing, and operating institutions for the mentally sick. In 1841, Dorothea Lynde Dix, in a report to the Massachusetts Legislature, boldly exposed the shameful conditions under which the insane of that commonwealth were being held. The sick were confined "in cages, closets, cellars, stalls, pens! Chained, naked, beaten with rods, and lashed into obedience!" [29] This was about fifty years after Philippe Pinel, leader in a revolution against the traditional method of handling mental patients, had removed the chains in the Parisian hospital Bicêtre.

While some of the responsible authorities and administrators of institutions distinguished themselves by their progressive attitude, others remained apathetic to the introduction of new practices. It was left to a victim of the deplorable conditions to mold public opinion. In 1908, Clifford Whittingham Beers described his own bitter experience in insane asylums and presented so eloquent a plea for a radical change that the civilized world was moved profoundly.[30] A wave of reforms spread. Beside the construction of functional buildings meeting modern hygienic standards, three factors became decisive in transforming a "house of horror" into a hospital inspiring confidence: the rise of psychiatry as a medical specialty, the general introduction of physical therapy and occupational therapy (in the widest sense of the term), and the development of new medical treatment methods that ended the era of therapeutic nihilism.

In an increasing number of communities the mental hospitals were staffed with competent, salaried personnel. In addition to physicians and nurses, other professional groups appeared more frequently on the payroll. In 1939, 176 dentists, 40 psychologists and psychometrists, 289 social workers, and 852 occupational therapists were employed full-time by state hospitals for mental disease. In the same year there was on the average 1 physician (excluding the superintendent) for every 245 patients in public hospitals—still considerably less than the standard ratio of not less than 1 physician to 150 patients, recommended by the American Psychiatric Association in 1926. The ratio of nurses and attendants was 1 for every 9 patients while the standard called for not less than 1 nurse for every 8 patients. Yet, only about 1 in 10 persons on the nursing staff of state hospitals for mental disease and only 1 in 20 of those doing nursing service in state institutions for the mentally defective were graduate nurses.[31] Obtaining experienced attendants of integrity and responsibility has remained a burning problem due to the inadequacy of both training opportunities and pay schedules.

A considerable number of the mental hospitals operated by public agencies rank high in quality. But there are also many institutions which are a disgrace to any community or government which calls itself civilized. Obsolete buildings, utterly insanitary conditions, a serious lack of competent nursing personnel, a paucity of psychiatrists, and a custodial atmosphere enveloping the whole institution are still frequently found. The history of mental hospitals is replete with instances where it took a scandal of major proportions to awaken public agencies to the need for drastic reforms. As G. W. F. Schlegel once remarked, "we learn from history that we learn nothing from history."

The turn to specialized services placing emphasis on medical treatment could not fail to change the function of the institution for the mentally sick. Facilities originally equipped to serve only patients with gross deviations now could be utilized also for those with slight anomalies. Instead of being preoccupied with rendering custodial care to incurable patients and segregating the antisocial sick, they could encourage early treatment and, thereby, function less as residential institutions. These opportunities have been recognized widely. In many countries "need of treatment," as proved by medical certificates, has been accepted as condition for hospitalization. Great Britain in 1930 legalized admission of patients for whom there was "prognosis of early recovery." All this meant that restoration of patients with remediable disorders to a useful life, if not full earning capacity, became a new and increasingly achieved objective of the mental hospital. Such shift in emphasis, however, created a new problem. As the average span of life increased and the number of old people rose, more patients with mental disorders related to advancing years were admitted. Their proportion in the hospital population tended to become larger. Is it inevitable that all these patients be accommodated in institutions? Is the modern mental hospital with its costly services, so urgently needed for treatment, the appropriate place for the institutionalization of patients with senile disorders?

The statutes governing admission to a mental hospital and the procedures followed in executing these laws have been adjusted to scientific progress in a few countries only. In the United States almost no formality was required before 1872. The legal requirements introduced since that year have proved to jeopardize the attainment of the very objectives for which the advocates of adequate

THE GROWTH OF PUBLIC HOSPITALS

service for the mentally sick have been fighting. The admission policies actually followed differ extremely in fundamentals as well as in details. According to Grover A. Kempf, nonjudicial and judicial methods are in use. The former include admission on the basis of voluntary application, certificate of a health officer, certificate of one physician, and certificate of more than one physician. In the latter group fall commitment by court or commission, both a survival of archaic practices that originated in misconception of the nature of mental deviation.[32]

The introduction of voluntary admission has been the bright spot in the development. It permitted application of early treatment and served to abate the evil reputation of the "madhouse." In the United States, Massachusetts became the pioneer in this movement in 1881. Yet sixty years later approximately one fourth of the states still had not followed suit. In Great Britain a nation-wide basis for the admission of voluntary patients has been created by legislation enacted in 1930, and in Sweden by the Mental Diseases Act of 1929, in force since 1931.

The number of patients receiving care in public facilities for the mentally sick and defective has been increasing steadily. Early figures are lacking. Recent data, however, indicate the general trend. In the period from 1931 to 1941 the mental hospital population as enumerated by the average census rose from 427,135 to 603,179, and the number of admissions jumped from 97,889 to 208,592. It must be noted that about 55 per cent of the total hospital population in 1941 were in facilities for the mentally sick and defective.

All but a few per cent of these patients are cared for in public facilities. This fact in itself does not necessarily indicate that they receive service free. But it does show the extent to which the public makes use of governmental institutions.

Public responsibility for the maintenance of mental patients in hospitals is acknowledged now much as it was in old times. The general tenor of early statutes in New England—mostly acts "for relieving idiots and distracted persons"—was to the effect that "insane persons, having no responsible relatives, [were] to be cared for by the town selectmen." In England, the local lunacy authorities, created in 1845, were charged with the duty of making provisions for all persons "certified as being of unsound mind and unable to pay for the care which they need." In Germany a nation-wide requirement to provide for the "indigent mentally sick and defective" in "appropriate institutions" was introduced in 1870.

As time went on, a tendency grew to interpret economic need in a more liberal way. Yet except in the case of serious mental illness the public institution was only for the indigent. This changed with the introduction of voluntary admission. The privilege was at first confined to patients able to pay for their care, but later extended to others in many states. Gradually the idea spread that the facilities and services of a public hospital should be available at fixed charges to anyone, regardless of his economic condition.

In the United States the patient's family usually contributes to the cost by paying such portion of the charges as it can afford, while tax funds are allotted to cover the deficit. In actual operation, however, fees are collected in only nineteen states.[33] The number of persons paying their charges in full has remained insignificant.

The revisions in admission policy are reflected in the income sheets of mental hospitals under government control. In 1935 payments from patients contributed on the average about 16 per cent of the total income; they ranged, by states, from less than 1 per cent to more than 60 per cent. Tax funds accounted for about 81 per cent on the average, ranging from less than 40 per cent to nearly 100 per cent.

Establishment and operation of a modern institution for persons with mental deviations go far beyond the needs and financial capacity of small political units. This discovery was made early and led to a break with the traditional policy of providing and administering facilities for the sick. One country after the other transferred the power and duty of establishing and maintaining mental hospitals from small units such as towns to larger ones such as counties, provinces, or states. In England county-wide organization was introduced in 1808. Before the war counties or county-boroughs provided nearly all beds in facilities for the mentally sick. In Germany since 1870 special administrative units covering parts or all of the territory of a state have been required to maintain mental hospitals, with the result that these authorities control the greater part of all available beds. In Sweden the national government is mainly responsible for mental hospitals. In 1940 it owned and operated institutions furnishing more than nine tenths of all beds for the mentally sick.

In the United States the states have come to occupy the leading position in this field. By 1940 all but one state operated one or more mental hospitals of their own. More than four fifths of all mental hospital beds were in state institutions serving a varying number of counties. Only about 8 per cent were in facilities maintained by counties or cities and a still smaller proportion, mainly serving veterans, was controlled by Federal agencies. All but 4 per cent of the patients institutionalized for mental defect and epilepsy were in state institutions.

GENERAL HOSPITALS

The principle of government responsibility for provision of adequate general hospitals, that is, hospitals receiving a variety of diseases, is undisputed. How far it should be applied is a matter of controversy in a score of countries. The basic issues in question are these: (1) Is establishment of general hospitals a legitimate function, if not a duty of government—just as the provision of schools, highways, sanitation, utilities, recreational facilities, and similar services essential for the welfare of the individual as well as the social organism? (2) Shall facilities built at public expense be operated for the benefit of all who want to use them or only for selected socio-economic groups? (3) If available to everybody, shall general hospitals maintained by public agencies charge self-supporting people for the use of the service at cost or in direct proportion to their ability to pay? (4) Where nongovernmental hospitals have developed, shall they be supervised by the state? Shall they be utilized and paid by public agencies for service to designated groups?

The broad policies followed by various countries in providing for general hospitals have differed sharply in the past. They have tended to become less dissimilar since about 1930. One group of countries, exemplified by the United States, Great Britain, and France, have relied on a general hospital system mainly supported by voluntary effort. A second group, of which the Scandinavian countries, Germany, and Austria are examples, have come to adopt a predominantly public system. A third group, exemplified by Russia, have decided to possess governmental hospitals only. In addition, a number of countries, including several in South America, have encouraged the establishment of hospitals by social insurance organizations.

The growth of general hospitals in the United States has been rapid. Paucity of information precludes a detailed analysis of the period prior to 1927. Beginning with that year more accurate data have been collected on the types of hospital service. More exact statistics on control of hospitals have been made available since 1934 and on general hospitals by type of control since 1938.

In 1942, general hospitals registered by the American Medical Association numbered 4,557 as against 4,322 in 1927. Facilities of this type have increased in number—although not without interruption—and exceed all others. In 1927 they constituted less than two thirds and in 1942 nearly three fourths of all registered hospitals. What is even more noteworthy, their bed capacity rose from 345,364 in 1927 to 594,260 in 1942. Striking, indeed, was this progress. But it was only part of a general and rapid advance in the entire hospital field. By 1942 the beds in general hospitals accounted for about 43 per cent of all, as compared with about 41 per cent in 1927, ranking second to those in mental and nervous hospitals. They were concentrated in densely populated regions, urban areas, and wealthier parts of the country. In agricultural states a large portion, if not the majority, of all general hospital beds were in the few urban centers.[34]

According to a 1939 survey of all facilities, registered and non-registered, the beds in general and other hospitals of similar type, excluding tuberculosis and mental hospitals, were available at the average rate of 3.83 per 1,000 population. The bed rate by states ranged from 1.57 to 7.13 per 1,000 population.[35] In other words, the state best supplied had four times as many beds per unit of population as the state ranking lowest. The majority of these hospitals were small. Nearly six tenths had less than 50 beds. If only the registered facilities are considered, nearly one fourth had fewer than 25 beds and another one fourth fell into the 25 to 49 beds category. Yet many of such small facilities, often ill-equipped, afforded the only hospital service in many a community.

How did the situation existing before the war compare with standards of quantitative adequacy? According to *The Need for a National Health Program*, 4.6 general hospital beds per 1,000 population, with a minimum of 2 beds for 1,000 population in rural areas, are necessary to meet essential needs.[36] The report of the American Medical Association for the year 1941 gave the average rate of general hospital beds (excluding the "allied" hospitals enumerated by the United States Bureau of the Census) as 4.1 per 1,000 population.

Even if one makes allowance for inaccuracies in reporting and inconsistencies in classifying hospitals, two general conclusions are well substantiated: despite the remarkable progress achieved in a relatively short period of time, the country as a whole is undersupplied with beds in general hospitals. Because of great disparity in the advance, the majority of the states fall below the standards suggested by experts.

It would mean ignoring a fundamental of hospital policy if emphasis were placed on the number rather than the quality of facilities. A substantial fraction of the general hospitals which are registered by the American Medical Association and a large proportion of the bed capacity in such facilities have been approved by the American College of Surgeons as meeting its minimum standards. According to the Council on Medical Education and Hospitals of the American Medical Association, "registration is a basic recognition, extended to all the hospitals and related institutions concerning which the Council has no evidence of irregular or unsafe practices." Approval by the American College of Surgeons means that the hospital meets a set of requirements fundamental to good hospital care. Facilities with fewer than 25 beds are excluded from consideration.

Voluntary effort must be given credit for most of the achievements in developing and improving the general hospital designed exclusively for the care of the sick. The pioneers in the field were physicians, often surgeons, who wanted a workshop in which to practice medicine; and nonprofit organizations, including many church-related organizations, which were founded to meet community needs.

The methods employed and the arguments advanced in promoting hospitals in the early days are of more than historical interest. When in the early seventeen fifties the Philadelphia physician Thomas Bond struggled hard to establish the first hospital exclusively for the care of the sick, it was the weight of Benjamin Franklin's influence that eventually tipped the scales in favor of the new idea. In his autobiography, Franklin made the following confession: "I do not remember any of my political manœuvres, the success of which gave me at the time more pleasure, or wherein, after thinking of it, I more easily excus'd myself for having made some use of cunning." When Samuel Bard in 1769 pleaded for the erection of a hospital in New York City, he emphasized that "the good effects of a Hospital" would not "be wholly confined to the poor, they would extend to every rank and greatly contribute to the safety and welfare of the whole community." Bard also was convinced that ". . . an institution of this nature . . . affords the best and only means of properly instructing pupils in the practice of medicine. . . ."[37]

Gradually the nonprofit general hospital came to occupy a dominant position. In 1941 the bed capacity in such facilities was approximately seven times as large as that in proprietary hospitals. On the other hand, the proprietary hospitals, mostly of small size, were numerous and important because they afforded the only hospital facility in many areas. Nongovernmental institutions furnished four out of five beds in general hospitals for community use.

Governments have contributed to the growth of general hospitals by encouraging and financially assisting voluntary efforts; and by establishing facilities of their own at local, state, and national level.

Financial assistance from public agencies for the construction, equipment, and improvement of voluntary general hospitals is a device tested by time and used widely. The Massachusetts General Hospital in Boston, begun in 1818 and opened in 1821, was financed by gifts from the will of two prominent citizens, subscriptions, and a substantial subsidy from the commonwealth. A recent example of the same principle, applied only to communities having needs created by the war, is the allocation of Federal funds for "defense public works," including hospitals.[38] More than half of the requests approved up to the end of 1942 came from voluntary hospitals planning to finance additions.

When cash on hand was scarce but some property available for disposal, public agencies not infrequently resolved to give aid in kind. Interesting examples of this method of supporting voluntary effort can be found in the history of Milwaukee, Wisconsin. In 1857 the municipality donated three acres of land out of the "Poor House property" to the Sisters of Charity of St. Vincent de Paul for a hospital which was completed in 1859 through gifts from citizens. In 1888, when some physicians set out to organize a hospital, the old central police station, erected in 1857, was "gratuitously" offered to the group.[39]

In developing general hospitals at public expense the various governmental agencies followed entirely different courses. Federal agencies established facilities for designated groups regardless of income and place of residence, but not for community use. Since the first marine hospitals were opened in 1802 to care for sick and disabled merchant seamen, the bed capacity under Federal control has grown substantially, and more groups have been declared eligible for service. In 1941 nearly 53 per cent of all general hospital beds maintained at public expense were in Federal facilities; they accounted for nearly one third of all public institutions for general service. Veterans constituted by far the largest single group of civilian patients hospitalized, and merchant seamen came next.[40]

Local and state governments, on the other hand, proceeded in an uncertain fashion. Most of them were unwilling to put money into general hospitals. If they did they wanted to provide for the sick poor residing in the area over which they had jurisdiction. The needs of the community were not considered at all in earlier times and only slightly since the turn of the nineteenth century.

In line with the old social philosophy which recognized destitution but not illness as a prerequisite for community action, governments turned to workhouses and almshouses in their search for facilities for the "reception" of the sick poor. These institutions were gradually equipped with special units for the ill. An early example of this policy is afforded by a measure adopted in the first half of the eighteenth century in South Carolina. The vestry of St. Philip's Parish was authorized by the governor to appropriate a piece of public land "whereon to erect proper buildings for the use of a Public Work-House and Hospital. . . ." In Great Britain the workhouse infirmary became one of the principal facilities for the hospitalization of poor persons. Shocking deficiencies in care aroused so much indignation that in 1865 the medical journal *The Lancet* branded them in an editorial with the telling title: "Our Workhouse Infirmaries: A National Scandal." Substantial improvements in building, equipment, staffing, and care were made later, but the system of retaining the sick poor in general mixed workhouses was discontinued only in the twentieth century.

Many a modern general hospital under public auspices had its origin in a workhouse. A typical example is the General Hospital, Vienna, now one of the leading municipal hospitals. In other instances, the public general hospital has grown from a workhouse and an isolation facility. The Bellevue Hospital of the City of New York dates back to a pesthouse erected in 1794 and a "Publick Workhouse and House of Correction," founded in 1736. At present it is a 2,800 bed general hospital, approved by the American College of Surgeons as meeting unconditionally its minimum standards, approved for training interns and for residencies by the American Medical Association, affiliated with leading medical schools, and operating an accredited school of nursing.

The institution of the poorhouse type also has played an important role in the history of the public hospital. The Boston Almshouse, erected in 1662, had a few beds for sick paupers—and that was all there was of public medical care facilities until early in the nineteenth century. Special provisions for the sick were scant in these institutions. Only slowly were sick rooms, wards, or infirmaries developed. There are communities in which such institutions fulfill the same function now as they did hundreds of years ago—to afford the only public service in a district for the sick without resources of their own. Many almshouses have continued to accommodate large numbers of patients with chronic illnesses, physical disabilities, and mental deviations, children as well as adults. They remind one of the sixteenth century concept of hospitals. Juan-Luis Vivès defined them as "places where the sick are fed and cared for, where a certain number of paupers is supported, where boys and girls are reared, where abandoned infants are nourished, where the insane are confined, and where the blind dwell."

In other instances, and they are many, the almshouse was the ancestor of a modern general hospital meeting high standards. Typical examples are the 2,300 bed Philadelphia General Hospital in Philadelphia, which originated in an almshouse opened in 1732; the 800 bed Grasslands Hospital in Valhalla, New York, a county hospital dating back to an early nineteenth century almshouse; and the Freedmen's Hospital in Washington, D.C., a 550 bed general hospital under control of the Federal government, which was opened in 1865 as a shelter for destitute refugees and freedmen and their wives and children.

In Great Britain the statutes and policies adopted after the passage of the Elizabethan Poor Law Act of 1601 insisted on maintenance of institutions of the poorhouse type to such an extent that prior to the great reform of 1929 hardly any public general hospitals were available for persons other than the poor.

The extent to which government participated in the provision of general hospitals in the United States cannot be stated for the period

THE GROWTH OF PUBLIC HOSPITALS

prior to 1938. The first fairly accurate enumeration, made in that year, gave the bed capacity in registered general hospitals under government control as 147,350 or 34.5 per cent of the total in registered general hospitals. By 1942, the number of such beds had risen to 291,766 and their proportion to 49.1 per cent. Nearly three fourths of all beds in publicly operated general hospitals were in facilities approved by the American College of Surgeons.[41]

At first glance the statistical data seem to indicate that the United States recently has steered in the direction taken before by many foreign countries: namely, toward the large-scale development of a tax-supported system of general hospitals for community use. Such is not the case. The greater part of the beds provided at public expense are available only to designated groups of individuals for whom the Federal government has assumed responsibility. By deducting these beds from the total in registered governmental facilities as given by the American Medical Association for the year 1942, a clearer picture is obtained. It appears that one in five general hospital beds was provided by city, county, state, and city-county facilities, in this order of frequency.

Before the war the beds maintained by public agencies were most numerous in states with high per capita income and concentrated in cities with populations of more than 100,000. Numerically and proportionately they declined rapidly outside of large urban areas. Only one seventh of all counties had a public general hospital. On the other hand, in a small number of counties the local governmental hospital was the only facility providing general hospital care. The beds furnished by general hospitals under government control represented approximately one third of all the general beds available in cities with populations of over 100,000 and approximately one fifth of those in less populous communities. Thus, the governmental general hospital was important only in a number of large cities and in a few rural areas.[42]

With the growth of public general hospitals a new and crucial problem has arisen: Who shall be admitted to a governmental facility?

One school of thought advances the idea that a hospital built at the expense of the taxpayer should be operated for the benefit of all who want its service; it should accept paying patients as well as those who could pay only part of their charges or nothing. There should be no class medicine. It would be incompatible with democratic ideals to maintain one set of hospitals exclusively for the poor and another for persons with resources of their own. Public hospitals accessible, attractive, and worthwhile to all would receive substantial income from paying patients, with the result that the deficit to be met by taxation would be reduced. They would effectively demonstrate the good use that can be made of tax funds and hereby stimulate community interest in demanding and supporting adequate health services in general.

This reasoning is sharply contested by a second school of thought. Public hospitals should admit only persons unable to afford care in private hospitals, if not solely "public charges." Strictly observed should be the principle of charity so admirably expressed in the words: "None may enter who can pay—none can pay who enters." Patients with resources of their own should be referred to nongovernmental hospitals. The entrance of government into this field would not be conducive to sound public policy. It would make unfair competition to the hard pressed voluntary hospitals and, in the long run, deal a mortal blow to such institutions.

In the United States until the end of the nineteenth century only the poor were accepted, and patients who paid anything were unknown in public general hospitals Since that time the admission policy has been liberalized in many sections of the country. Patients able to pay hospitalization costs in full or in part are admitted. On the whole, their proportion is small, negligible in large cities, somewhat greater outside urban centers, and substantial only in a number of localities where special conditions prevail. The Quincy City Hospital in Massachusetts, which accepts any patients being treated by the physicians on the staff, reported in 1939 that three fourths of the sick cared for were private patients.[43]

On the other hand, in some parts of the country laws or charters prevent hospitals maintained by city, county, or state from accepting "pay" patients, with the result that the public facilities often are inadequately occupied while the others are overcrowded. An illustration of this policy is afforded by the "Act concerning the admission of applicants to state supported charity hospitals . . ." adopted in Louisiana in 1926. This law states that "it shall be the duty of the Board of Administrators of the State Charity Hospital, or hospitals supported by the State, to refuse admission for treatment to persons

THE GROWTH OF PUBLIC HOSPITALS

not poor and destitute; provided that in no case shall persons of any description be refused emergency treatment. . . ." [44] In California a court decision handed down in 1936 prohibited the admission to county hospitals of patients who "either themselves or through legally responsible relatives, can provide themselves with equally efficient care and treatment in private institutions." [45]

In Great Britain until 1929 the public hospitals were restricted to persons who might be considered as destitute. Persons entering such an institution were automatically classified as paupers. These conditions have been removed since, and private blocks or wings have been increasingly added to public facilities. In a score of other foreign countries it has long been established public policy to make the service of a governmental hospital available to everybody.

The number of patients who receive care in general hospitals maintained by local, state, and Federal governments in the United States has been growing steadily. Moreover, public facilities have increasingly shared in the total amount of service rendered by general hospitals.

In 1941, the registered general hospitals under government control reported 3,197,417 admissions or about 30 per cent of a total of 10,646,947. In 1938, when the first more accurate compilation was made, they cared for 2,170,189 admissions or 25.4 per cent of a total of 8,545,930. Of the general hospital population, as enumerated by the average census, 44.1 per cent (160,128 persons) were in governmental facilities in 1941, as compared with 39.1 per cent (114,627 persons) in 1938. These figures indicate that hospitalization in public facilities has come to play an important role. However, it must be remembered that a substantial fraction of the public general hospitals are Federal facilities operated for the benefit of selected groups in the population. The extent to which the "average citizen" is hospitalized in public facilities can be estimated from the figures published by the American Medical Association. In 1941 approximately every fifth patient admitted to general hospitals received service in a city, county, state, or city-county facility, in that order; and about one fourth of the general hospital population, as enumerated by the daily census, was in these facilities.

The public hospitals which are open to the general public charge "pay" patients for the service rendered. They depend on tax funds, and occasionally also on other sources of income, to cover the remaining costs of operation.[46] It is interesting to note that in some foreign countries, primarily Sweden, the charges are kept low, frequently at one fourth or less of the actual costs, so as to make hospitalization readily accessible.

Where the great majority of the hospitalized sick come from the ranks of those accepted for public assistance, the income sheet of the public hospital shows insignificant amounts received from patients. Where self-supporting people from all walks of life avail themselves of the service offered, a substantial part of the hospital income is derived from patient payments. In 1935, when some degree of recovery from the depths of the depression had been achieved, the registered general and allied hospitals controlled by local agencies of government received 14.4 per cent of their revenues from patients and 83.6 per cent from taxes. The larger hospitals had a relatively higher income from taxes than facilities with less than 50 beds.[47] However, in those areas in which a public hospital constituted the only registered community facility for general or special service for acute illness, the situation was reversed. Patient payments accounted for 76.1 per cent, tax funds for 21.4 per cent, and other sources for 2.5 per cent of the hospital income.[48] A study of 247 hospitals in cities with populations of less than 100,000 showed that 45 per cent recorded, in 1938, receipts from patients which equalled three fourths or more of the expenditure, and about two thirds covered half or more of their current expenses by income from paying patients.[49]

The costs of building, equipping, and operating a general hospital worthy of the name have risen continuously and sharply since the time when a boardinghouse for sick people was all that was needed. Even a few decades ago when these costs were a fraction of what they are now, small political units in general and districts with low per capita income in particular found it hard, if not impossible, to support the establishment of anything but a small, ill-equipped facility. They could barely afford to pay the charges made by nongovernmental hospitals for care rendered to the indigent. Larger political units also often had considerable difficulties in raising the money necessary for the building of a good hospital of moderate or large size.

Countries which were anxious to develop an adequate hospital system fully recognized that the problem was national in scope. They adjusted their public policy accordingly. The responsibility for public hospitals was distributed between various levels of government. Local authorities were charged with providing, operating, and administering general hospitals. Central agencies were made responsible for directing, coordinating, guiding, supervising, and financially assisting the work of local agencies. In many instances, financial and administrative responsibility at the local level was transferred from small communities to large units, such as cities, counties, or provinces. They were authorized, and in a number of instances required, to provide adequate general hospitals according to need and to operate them in conformity with general rules laid down by the central authority. The state or national government made substantial grants-in-aid to local agencies. The state only or state and locality jointly maintained teaching hospitals.

The following examples of foreign developments may serve to illustrate these points. As early as 1806 the King of Denmark issued an "Order in Council" that each county should have one to three hospitals according to local needs. In England the Local Government Act of 1929 transferred responsibility for health services from the multiple small authorities to larger units, the county councils and county-borough councils, gave them power to provide general hospitals for community use, and provided for grants-in-aid from the national government. In France the national government in 1932 allocated funds to stimulate the erection of new general hospitals at the local level. In Sweden the Hospital Act of 1940 vested responsibility for general hospitals in the provincial councils which were given vast powers.

In the United States it was mostly cities and counties and in a few instances states (primarily Louisiana, Mississippi, and Pennsylvania) that assumed responsibility for general hospitals for community use. A considerable number of states, however, established state university hospitals. Federal participation has been sporadic and on a very limited scale. Funds of the Public Works Administration and the Works Progress Administration and allocations provided by the Community Facilities Act of 1941 have been used for new constructions, additions, and improvements.

Failure to initiate a nation-wide hospital policy based on the principle of Federal-state cooperation has resulted in a serious lack of adequate facilities in many parts of the country and in the perpetuation of needless and wasteful rivalry between governmental and nongovernmental hospitals.

UNSOLVED PROBLEMS

The increase and expansion of public facilities for the care of the sick in the United States has taken place without over-all planning. The result is that two major shortcomings have come to the fore. Hospital beds, both general and special, are very unevenly distributed. They are relatively numerous in wealthy areas and rare in poor sections of the country. Furthermore, governmental and nongovernmental activities in the hospital field are uncoordinated. They duplicate in some communities and are entirely lacking in others. These facts clearly prove the need for a hospital policy devised, accepted, and carried out by all groups concerned.

The moment has come to attain a functional coordination of all existing hospitals meeting modern standards, regardless of ownership. The time is here to substitute concerted for isolated effort.

· 3 ·

FROM "FREE DISPENSARY" TO PUBLIC MEDICAL CENTER

WHEN the first "dispensaries" in the English-speaking world began operation in the eighteenth century, "relief of the sick poor" was their primary objective and private support their only method of finance. When, in the thirties and forties of the twentieth century, plans were laid for the future organization of medical care, an entirely different approach to the clinic problem was urged. Representative groups and agencies in several countries recommended that the practice of medicine for the whole population be conducted through a system of "medical centers" or "health centers" as the basis of group practice. Such facilities were to be established out of tax funds. What began as isolated charity service for the poor has thus grown to be regarded as an integral part of modern health policy for all of the people.

At present a variety of facilities ranging from a primitive room to elaborate functional buildings are lumped together under the general term clinic. All of them are designed for ambulatory service. But they differ sharply in general objectives, type of service offered, administrative organization, and group of people served.

Clinics may be divided into two broad categories: those which have been initiated and developed as nonprofit institutions under the auspices of public agencies and voluntary organizations, and those which have been set up by groups of physicians for the purpose of practicing medicine ("private group clinics").

The nonprofit clinics are of two basically different types. One set is organized primarily to provide treatment for the ambulatory sick belonging to certain economic groups, and a second set is organized primarily to preserve and promote the health of apparently well persons by providing for diagnostic services, health education, and health supervision. In neither case is the distinction between treatment and preventive services fully maintained. Exceptions to the rule are made in a few areas of health activities where the need for integration has been felt most. In contrast, the group clinics maintained by physicians in private practice are organized to offer service without distinction as to type. The need of the patient and his ability to pay are the principal factors determining the scope of care supplied.

From the standpoint of administrative organization the facility which is part of a hospital—the out-patient department—can be distinguished from the "unattached" institution. Such a facility may have a varying number of divisions for general and specialists' services, each called a clinic, or it may be limited to one particular type of service.

The differences in the general objectives of the various types of clinics are reflected in the policies and procedures governing admission. The great majority of the treatment clinics are maintained for recipients of public assistance, general and special, and, to a varying extent, also for people who cannot afford such service at private rates. A relatively small number are operated for the benefit of other selected groups, such as industrial workers and university students. A few are designed for service to the whole community. Clinics of the preventive type are open either to anyone who wants to use them or to persons below a certain income level. The services of private group clinics are available to the public at large regardless of income, although in actual operation self-supporting people above the low-income level constitute the vast majority of all patients treated.

How, then, did it happen that clinics with so different functions for so differing socio-economic groups evolved? The answer to this question will be found by tracing the development of the various types of clinics.

TREATMENT CLINICS

Treatment clinics were the first to be established. Originally their primary function was the "dispensing" of free drugs, with medical attention playing a minor role. Hence the name "dispensary." The interdependence of clinic and hospital care was realized early. The Philadelphia Dispensary, founded in 1786 as the first of its kind in the United States, regarded as its principal object "to afford relief to the poor in those cases where removal to a public hospital would, for any approved reason, be ineligible." That even the best clinic service could meet but part of the needs of the sick also was fully recognized from the very beginning. Home care was included in the scope of service. The second oldest treatment clinic, the New York Dispensary (founded in 1791), assured its patients that those "who are not well enough to come to the dispensary will be visited at their respective places of abode"; and the Boston Dispensary, the third oldest (founded in 1796), stated: "The sick without being pained by a Separation from their Families may be attended and relieved in their own Houses."

In a later phase of the development the emphasis on various types of services shifted markedly. More and more efforts were directed toward provision of "medical and surgical aid," although distribution of drugs and some appliances, free of charge or at low rates, continued to be an important function. Home care was provided less and less, in many instances given up and in other instances confined to emergency cases. The dispensary became in fact a clinic for ambulatory patients.

The decisive turn in the evolution of treatment clinics occurred in the twentieth century. Since the second decade such facilities have rapidly increased in number. What is even more important, they have been devised, organized, and operated in new ways.

The concept gained ground that the clinic was the appropriate instrument to attain quality, efficiency, convenience, and economy of service for patients who were not bedridden. The conviction spread that well-organized clinic service could contribute much to the proper and economical utilization of hospital beds by determining indications for hospitalization, caring for patients who would otherwise be hospitalized, and providing for aftercare and follow-up of discharged patients where needed. And there was agreement on the potential value of well-equipped and well-staffed clinics to teaching and research.

As these ideas crystallized, the organization of clinics was adapted to the new objectives. Following the original policy many organizations continued to develop facilities which were not a division of a hospital. This was done chiefly when special groups, such as industrial workers or college and university students, were served; when private physicians practiced as a group; when a system of district health service was developed; and when adequate hospitals were not within easy travel distance. The number of such "unattached" treatment clinics grew remarkably. But not less notable was a trend to make the facility for the treatment of the ambulatory sick a unit of a facility for "in-patients." Most of the general and special hospitals began to render some service to ambulatory patients, but only a relatively small number developed an organized service with regularly scheduled hours.

The first fairly accurate study, made in 1936 as part of the National Health Inventory, indicated that 769 hospitals, mainly of the general type, maintained fully organized out-patient departments, while many more provided for some out-patient service.[1] Half of them had been opened after 1920, a fourth during the twenty years preceding that date, and the remainder before 1900. Out-patient departments have been primarily a large-city development. By 1940 such facilities, varying in number as well as in quality, existed in almost all the larger cities, in about half of the cities of 50,000 population, but only sporadically in communities with less than 10,000 population and in rural areas. Although there is reason to assume that some progress has been made since, three facts have remained essentially unchanged: the existence of out-patient departments at only one in about six general hospitals; the scarcity of such facilities outside large cities and their lack in small communities; and the concentration of the existing clinics in a few geographic regions, primarily in the states along the Northern and Middle Atlantic seaboard and in the region of the Great Lakes.

Aware of the significance of the clinic movement, private organizations and governmental agencies took steps to direct the development into proper channels. The American Hospital Association, endorsing proposals worked out by its Committee on Out-Patient Work, adopted ideals and policies for out-patient work.[2] The American College of Surgeons took active part in the development of minimum standards.[3] A growing number of states made the operation of clinics subject to license.

Most of the out-patient departments operating at regularly scheduled hours receive any type of disease. Some provide service without scheduling regular specialty periods, others have organized divisions and subdivisions equipped and staffed to give specialists' care. This trend toward departmentalization has become more marked in recent times. Most frequently found at present are divisions of general medical service; general surgery; pediatrics; obstetrics and gynecology; and eye, ear, nose, and throat diseases. Many of the larger treatment clinics have been subdivided to such an extent that a vast range of special services is available in a community.

To give an example, the out-patient clinics maintained by a number of hospitals in Rochester, New York, provide a large variety of specialized services through the following main divisions: medicine, general; medicine, special (with nineteen specialties represented); surgery, general; surgery, special (with thirteen categories); obstetrics and gynecology; pediatrics; psychiatry; dentistry; ancillary services such as X-ray and physical therapy; and tuberculosis.[4]

With the increase and continuous improvement of their resources in equipment and personnel treatment clinics could expand their field of activity to perform functions formerly not envisaged.

Diagnostic, specialist, and consultant services at the request of practicing physicians were additions that were willingly offered and gladly accepted in some communities.

Teaching of medical students and physicians, of student and graduate nurses, and of social workers in training and after graduation was developed with increasing frequency although not on a large scale. Realization that a clinic could be an important adjunct to the theoretical education and hospital instruction of medical students had been one of the factors influencing the early development of teaching clinics in connection with medical schools. Now the educational value of clinics in general was recognized and enhanced by the extension of teaching opportunities to more professional groups. Research not only in clinical subjects but on illness in its socio-economic setting was taken up here and there.

Occasionally public clinics were charged with the medical examination of all applicants for relief who claimed disability and with the provision of rehabilitation service where it was indicated.

By far the most significant development—and one of fundamental importance—was the expansion of treatment clinics into the field of preventive health work. Immunization and vaccination as well as health examinations and regular health supervision of apparently healthy children and adults were increasingly provided, and regular preventive clinic sessions were conducted in out-patient departments.

The treatment clinic, once a place where general practitioners rendered some service to sick people, thus has reached a significant stage in its evolution. It is beginning to develop into a highly organized and departmentalized center for the distribution of a large variety of such services as are essential to the prevention, cure, and mitigation of illness.[5]

Treatment clinics set up as nonprofit institutions operate on the basis of definite eligibility requirements.

The original dispensaries were strictly for persons "unable by reason of poverty to procure" drugs and medical attention. Usually eligibility was restricted to the "worthy" poor. The noble spirit guiding the founders of some of the early dispensaries is well exemplified in the declaration of purposes of the Boston Dispensary: "Those who have seen better Days may be comforted without being humiliated; and all the Poor receive the Benefits of a Charity the more refined, as it is the more secret." Gradually the admission policy was liberalized as the mounting costs of good medical care and profound socio-economic changes combined to multiply the number of persons in need of aid. More and more clinics accepted self-supporting people who could not afford the services of specialists and the costs of expensive tests, treatment methods, and drugs at private rates.

To facilitate the determination of the patient's ability to pay, the American Hospital Association recommended the following procedure:

In determining the admission of individual cases to an out-patient clinic, three factors need to be considered with due consideration of local community conditions; namely, the income of the patient or family, the size and responsibilities of the family according to a reasonable standard of living, and the character and probable cost of adequate medical treatment for the disease or condition found.[6]

Reconciling the desire to help the sick in need with the determination not to encroach on the field of the private physician proved to be a task beset with great difficulties. Working arrangements have been reached but they are not uniform. Anxious not to burn the candle at both ends, some clinics ordinarily admit for treatment only patients accepted for public assistance and those referred by physicians in the community or recognized social agencies. Others regularly extend their service to "medically needy" persons according to interpretations that vary widely depending upon the community setup. Financial eligibility is not considered, however, if patients are referred by physicians in private practice for diagnosis or special treatment. In actual operation, recipients of public assistance constitute the large majority of clinic clients. It is due to this fact that in public opinion the word clinic has continued to carry a charity connotation, if not a "connotation of indigency." Significantly, periods of high employment and earnings markedly decrease the number of persons who demand and receive service, leaving mainly the very young and the very old, the chronically sick, and the physically and mentally disabled under the care of clinics.

Clinics organized for special groups operate on principles basically different from those observed by institutions for the needy. Employment, rather than inability to pay, serves to determine eligibility for service established in industry. Enrollment, rather than financial need, makes those attending colleges and universities eligible for the student health service maintained by the institution.

The trend to relax eligibility requirements was accompanied by a tendency to differentiate between free clinics and others where patients were charged small amounts. This constituted a departure from the old tradition of free service dating back to a time when only very poor persons were admitted. Many patients now were not only able to contribute something to the costs of their care but took a pride in paying a modest sum. The costs of operating clinics had increased to such an extent that new sources of revenue had to be found. Apart from these considerations clinic administrators attached importance to the psychological fact that any "gratuitous offer" is looked on with distrust.

In 1925 the Committee on Out-Patient Work of the American Hospital Association recommended that "stated fees be charged to patients for admission, and that additional charges be made for medicines, appliances, and other special procedures or materials." [7]

This recommendation has been followed widely although not uniformly. At present the general policy as well as the fee schedule varies greatly, even within the same area. Some clinics, primarily those under government control, make no or only nominal charges and have remained essentially "free" clinics. Others request payment in the form of an—often graded—admission fee. Still others make charges (from twenty-five cents to one dollar and more) for each visit; for certain services such as laboratory and X-ray tests, drugs, appliances, and physiotherapy; or for both.

The majority of patients pay little although conditions vary widely. For instance, the out-patient department of the Mountainside Hospital in Montclair, New Jersey, reported that 51 per cent of the white and 39 per cent of the Negro patients paid the full charge in 1939.[8] Usually income from fees covers only a minor part of the expenditures for the service. A study of 174 out-patient departments in 1936 indicated that governmental institutions defrayed about 15 per cent and nongovernmental institutions more than 40 per cent of their expenditures by income from patients' fees.[9]

Before the war the actual costs of out-patient service, excluding compensation of physicians, were estimated at seventy-five cents to one dollar a visit in facilities providing good quality of care. Fairly typical is the experience in Rochester, New York. The Rochester Hospital Council estimated the average cost of each out-patient visit at ninety-five cents during the fiscal year ending March, 1940, while the income received from patients averaged thirty-eight cents per visit. The out-patient department of the New Haven Hospital in Connecticut, a teaching clinic affiliated with the Yale School of Medicine, covered approximately one fifth of its expenses in 1940 through patients' fees, and the Hartford Dispensary in Connecticut, an unattached clinic, received about one fourth of its total income in 1941 from payments by patients.

The mere fact that clinics are available in industry or institutions of higher learning does not imply that they can be used free of charge. In a number of instances all or a varying number of services are provided without cost to the individual. In other instances payment must be made according to special arrangements, widely varying in type.

Private initiative has created treatment clinics in the United States. Voluntary organizations were principally responsible for their development until about the middle of the nineteenth century and held a dominant place in the field until about 1930. Since that time local, state, and Federal agencies of government have shared responsibility with voluntary organizations on a larger scale. Originally they had confined their efforts to providing simple unattached dispensaries. There was always some space in a public building that could be utilized for health services—even if it were only a room next door to the sheriff's office or a dark corner in the basement of the police department. Later a tendency came to the fore to create functional buildings.

The number of unattached tax-supported clinics has increased mainly since the turn of the century. But the greater advance occurred along an entirely different line. More and more emphasis was placed on utilization of hospital resources in personnel and equipment by developing clinics attached to hospitals.

Of 769 out-patient departments studied in 1936 about one fourth were in government controlled facilities, mainly in general hospitals and frequently in tuberculosis hospitals.[10] While the nongovernmental institutions were leading in point of numbers, those under government control were responsible for nearly half of the volume of service rendered. Subsequently in many areas visits to voluntary institutions tended to decline further while those to public clinics were increasing.

Out-patient departments in hospitals under government control not only provide much of the care for the needy but render their services largely at public expense. A study of 174 out-patient departments in 1936 revealed that slightly more than 85 per cent of the income of governmental units was derived from tax-funds as against only 4 per cent in the case of nongovernmental facilities.[11]

In recent years the old idea of unattached treatment clinics has been revived in modern form. Public policy is beginning to recognize that a new approach to the organization of medical service, both curative and preventive, is necessary.

In a number of instances public agencies have assumed responsibility for the establishment of centers in communities in great need of medical service. These facilities are designated for use by all residents rather than just the needy, equipped according to modern standards, staffed with full-time personnel, and intended for preventive as well as treatment service. Their construction and equipment are financed out of tax funds, while the costs of medical care are defrayed largely, if not exclusively, by organized prepayments of all those who agree to participate in a program of voluntary health insurance. This implies that membership in a prepayment plan rather than medical or financial need determines whether or not a person is eligible to receive service when needed.

The combination of tax support for the establishment of essential facilities and of insurance for the payment of certain services has been applied in various parts of the country. It has been used by the Farm Security Administration in about forty resettlement projects for low-income farmers; by local housing authorities in cooperation with the California Physicians' Service for the tenants of public housing projects in a few places on the West Coast; and by the Tennessee Valley Authority for its construction workers and their dependents, and also for other residents, in about ten rural areas. In all these instances the public clinic is conceived as the hub around which all community health activities, curative and preventive, revolve.

In the Soviet Union tax-supported clinics for treatment as well as for preventive work are being developed systematically.[12] In some other foreign countries they are established primarily to meet the needs of rural areas. Chile and Peru have built them to render ambulatory care to all persons covered by social insurance.

PREVENTIVE CLINICS

Preventive clinics owe their development to the recognition that the principles of early diagnosis by organized case-finding and periodic health examinations, of health guidance, and of systematic medical and social follow-up can best be attained by the establishment of centers properly equipped and staffed for such a complex task.

A large variety of clinic services for the prevention of illness and preservation and promotion of good health have come into existence since the movement started with the introduction of the tuberculosis clinic in Great Britain (Sir Robert Philip in Edinburgh, 1887) and of the well-baby conference, primarily in France (Pierre-Constant Budin, in 1892). In the United States preventive health services have been established more frequently since the turn of the century and have developed rapidly since 1920. Their growth in type as well as in number has been greatly accelerated by Federal participation in public health work since 1935.

A systematic classification of the multitude of clinic services commonly referred to as preventive is hard to make. Only those are considered here which are organized on the basis of a continuing program, with physicians or dentists conducting scheduled sessions at regular intervals.

The preventive clinics rendering organized individual service may be divided, according to the lines of approach they use, into two broad categories: those serving groups of apparently well persons who due to age, sex, occupation, or socio-economic conditions are exposed to health dangers; and those designated especially for persons suffering with or suspected of and exposed to a specified disease or group of closely related diseases.

In the first category maternal and infant, preschool child, and school child health services are outstanding, although their relative frequency varies greatly not only from country to country but from one area to another within the same country. Services for youths and adults are infrequent; if organized, they are mainly provided for students attending institutions of higher learning and for groups of industrial workers that are exposed to specific work hazards.

Among the services focused on prevention of certain diseases or conditions, the tuberculosis, venereal disease, and immunization clinics account for the large majority. Those for dental diseases and defects, orthopedic conditions, eye diseases and defects, mental deviations, and malignant tumors make up most of the rest.

The total number of facilities to which the term "preventive clinic" can be justly applied and the extent to which selected types of clinic service are provided in the United States at present are unknown. No attempt has been made to obtain a composite picture of all provisions of this type through nation-wide reporting based on exact definition and proper classification.

A study of ninety-four selected counties in 1936 showed that both the number of preventive clinics and the variety of services offered were relatively largest in densely settled counties.[13] It is certain that substantial progress has been made since that time, but the inadequacy of the existing services is admittedly still very great.

A student of the subject who in the absence of accurate data tried to obtain an impression of the over-all picture by traveling crisscross through the country would have no difficulty in arriving at five major conclusions. (1) Areas outside of large cities in general and communities with less than 20,000 population in particular are grossly undersupplied; rural areas are very rarely provided with the most essential preventive clinic services. (2) There are areas where within a radius of one hundred miles many communities point with pride to a large number and great variety of high-grade preventive clinic services, while other districts have only primitive, if any, provisions. (3) The services actually available even in the most intensely promoted fields of activity fall short of quantitative standards. (4) Even in the most advanced regions the preventive clinic program is far from being balanced, emphasizing and often unnecessarily duplicating selected services while neglecting others equally essential to both the individual and the community. (5) The quality of the various provisions differs immensely.

The basic functions of preventive clinics include the following: (1) examination by competent professional personnel for the purpose of establishing a diagnosis either of physical and mental fitness or of sickness; (2) information, advice, and guidance of the individual or groups of individuals as to health and related socio-economic, occupational, and psychological problems; (3) consultation service to physicians in private practice and to public and recognized private agencies; (4) home visits for case-finding, follow-up, and home care; and (5) coordination of diagnostic and educational activities with treatment services and social work. However, great disparity prevails in the emphasis placed upon the various functions. Neither all the clinics offering similar services nor the various types of clinics follow the same practices.

One of the most interesting attempts to broaden preventive health activities and bring them into close relation with social work was made in England. The Pioneer Health Centre at Peckham (South London), opened in 1926, was designed to study the physiological and psychological conditions of a large unselected group of urban families by observing all aspects of their life and all their various relationships in the social setting of the Centre, to investigate what in fact constitutes good health, how far it is enjoyed, and what measures can be taken to prevent the deterioration of the health of an individual.[14]

Well-organized and properly conducted diagnostic and educational clinic services intensify existing desire and create new demand for medical care in general and for specialists' care and special treatment methods in particular. Many persons are discovered and encouraged to seek treatment who have been unaware of an illness or defect, uncertain about the nature of a "trouble," or inclined to belittle a condition. However, diagnosis and education are only means to an end. Early, competent, and thorough treatment must be received where indicated. How else would it be possible to attain the objective of public health, defined by C.-E. A. Winslow as "the production of a nation of men and women and children possessed of vitality and effectiveness and happiness." [15] The question then immediately arises: If the facilities and personnel available for the care of the sick are not adequate both in quality and quantity, and if the costs of good care cannot be afforded by the patient, how can preventive clinics function effectively?

In the first phase of their development preventive clinics were operated on the premise that prevention and cure are two distinct arts. It was a settled policy to refer patients needing treatment to a private physician if resources were available or to a treatment center for free or low-cost care if financial need was established.

Experience soon proved how difficult it was in practice to determine the boundary between prevention and treatment, although the necessity of such a dividing line for administrative purposes was fully recognized. It was noticed that many of the people attending preventive clinics had trifling disorders or needed minor services for which they ordinarily did not seek medical attention even if urged. It became more and more evident that the control of certain diseases was seriously impeded by the separation of preventive and curative services. Taking cognizance of these facts one group of preventive clinics began to treat borderline conditions and to provide for such "minor dispensary services" as were not otherwise readily available. Well-baby clinics often took over the management of nutritional disorders. School clinics dressed simple wounds and treated certain skin diseases. Orthopedic clinics furnished casts and braces. Other clinics added specific treatment to their basic functions. In many countries the tuberculosis clinics provided pneumothorax treatment, usually refill service, for all needy patients and those referred by private practitioners for this purpose. More than one third of the tuberculosis clinics in the United States have adopted this policy. Still other clinics developed into centers where corrective services were not less emphasized than examination, consultation, and health guidance. Typical examples are the venereal disease and dental clinics which accept for treatment such patients as meet the—widely varying—eligibility requirements.

The trend from limited to inclusive provisions in foreign countries is strikingly illustrated by the development of the British school health service. In 1907 compulsory health examination of school children was introduced. When it became apparent that the needs for medical care were not adequately met by the traditional referral method, the local authorities were required by law to provide for curative services. To discharge this duty the public agencies established school clinics, including medical, dental, and orthopedic treatment clinics, and staffed them with salaried physicians. Before the war England and Wales possessed more than two thousand such services, operated at nominal or no charges according to the economic conditions of the parents.

A large number of preventive clinics are housed in out-patient departments of hospitals. This form of organization, it was thought, would offer many advantages. Available space, equipment, and personnel may be utilized profitably. The preventive services may be closely related to those for the ambulatory sick; the work of out-patient departments may be integrated with that of the hospital; and the hospital, thus, may become a true health center. But to pass beyond the stage of a beautiful theory proved to be difficult.

Among the many obstacles to the integration of the various services, two stood out as formidable: the inadequate allocation of experienced professional personnel for out-patient and preventive health service, and the division of authority over the various facilities and activities. Moreover, it has been realized that problems other than the adoption of sound administrative practices deserve most careful consideration. Hospitals of good quality are scarce, if not lacking, in many areas. Often, they are located at considerable distance from the districts where people of moderate or small means live. If frequent time-and-money-consuming rides must be made to reach a preventive clinic many people are likely to think twice before they avail themselves of the opportunity offered. Distance and inadequate transportation can easily defeat the purpose of bringing the service directly to the people.

Aware of the difficulties involved in the use of out-patient departments, official as well as nongovernmental agencies increasingly turned to the provision of preventive services in special units outside of hospitals and in close proximity to the center of the population to be served.

With the growing specialization of preventive health activities a large variety of "single-type" clinics were introduced, and a new problem arose. The functional and administrative coordination of all local health activities became imperative. While there was general agreement about the objectives, much controversy arose about the best method of accomplishing the desired end.[16]

The "all-under-one-roof" principle appeared not only to be applicable to the organization of preventive health services but to hold great promise if put to proper use. The people attending clinics would find it more convenient, time-conserving, and money-saving to obtain various services at one place and in the course of one visit. The specialists in charge of various divisions would be able to cooperate with each other more intensively and more extensively. The time of professional and clerical personnel would be utilized in a more economical way. The administrative work of various agencies would be centralized, correlated, relieved of duplication and overlapping and, thereby, simplified.

Out of such considerations grew the concept of the "district health center." This facility, according to Haven Emerson "as inevitable as the district fire house, school or police station," [17] embodies two ideas: decentralization of direct service by local horizontal organization, and concentration of competent professional personnel, special equipment, and administrative activities. It houses a variety of clinics and also certain bureaus for the administration of health work within a district. Ordinarily it is not affiliated with a hospital.

Many students of the subject believe that complete community health centers should be built around hospitals rather than as separate units detached from facilities for the care of the sick. The present policy reflects the profound disagreement over the function of the district health center. One school of thought holds that only the various services provided by official health agencies should be coordinated in a center.[18] Another school of thought maintains that "all of the public and private health, welfare and relief agencies working in a district" should be grouped together under one roof.[19] Illustrations of the various approaches used are afforded by the health centers in Boston, Massachusetts; New York City; Buffalo, New York; Wilkes-Barre, Pennsylvania; Alameda County and Los Angeles County, California; and Washington, D.C.

The total number of true district health centers in actual operation is small, but the idea has fallen on fertile soil in a score of countries and is likely to be translated into practice more frequently in the future in connection with the reorganization of medical service.

If specialized service is to reach the large number of families living in thinly settled regions, small towns, and rural communities, the organization must be adapted to the particular conditions. Where people ordinarily cannot come to the clinic because of the distances and cost of travel, the clinic must come to the people.

Clinics "on wheels" have been increasingly put into service to make a circuit of designated points throughout a state, or its larger political subdivisions, and hold sessions at each place according to a prearranged schedule. Such traveling clinics are primarily used to carry out programs for the prevention of physical handicaps among children, to make routine roentgenological examinations for tuberculosis, to provide dental care, and to furnish services needed for the control of venereal disease. In the United States a number of state agencies employ such mobile units.

The nation-wide application of this principle for the X-ray examination of every resident is contemplated by the National Association for the Campaign against Tuberculosis in Sweden. There, at the end of 1942, a series of special motor busses with laboratories capable of making 100 X-ray photographs an hour were under construction.

In trying to formulate appropriate policies and procedures governing the admission to preventive clinics both the sponsoring agencies and the professions concerned found themselves in a dilemma. On the one hand all agreed on the objectives and the urgent need of promoting preventive services. On the other hand, opinions clashed not only on the principle of using clinics for such purpose but on the best method by which a dividing line could be drawn between clinic activities and private practice.

One school of thought maintained that the effectiveness of preventive services depended upon the time at which action was taken, the completeness with which groups essential to the building of a healthy nation were reached, and the period over which the individuals belonging to such groups remained under regular health supervision and guidance. This task was clearly beyond the ability of an individual physician to accomplish. The clinic with its special provisions for finding, holding, and following up individuals in need of health protection was well equipped to "do the job," and ought to impose no restrictions on admission so as to accomplish the end desired by all. A second group, though endorsing the principle of clinic service, urged that only people below the comfort level or only those unable to pay a private physician be admitted. A third group wished "to have the family doctor take care of his patients in health as well as in time of illness" and to have the doctor's office become a health center.[20]

Wrestling with this intricate problem and trying to interpret the situation in an objective, open-minded, and sympathetic way, all agreed that no perfect solution could be found so long as the physicians depended on fees from patients for their livelihood. However, understandings between the health agencies promoting clinic service and the physicians in private practice became the rule rather than the exception.

In general a tendency appeared to rank the principle of prevention first and economic considerations last. The recognition grew that there was a wide-spread need for preventive clinic services; that a large fraction of the population was unable to pay and an even larger proportion not accustomed to seek private physicians' advice when in apparently good health. Liberal admission policies for preventive clinics were increasingly emphasized.

The National Tuberculosis Association, in its *Tuberculosis Clinic Manual*,[21] recommended that the clinic's "facilities for *diagnosis* should be free to all who care to take advantage of its benefits." The majority of the tuberculosis clinics follow this policy.[22] The United States Public Health Service suggested the abandoning of the practice of admitting to venereal disease clinics only those patients who had been referred by private physicians.[23]

As a general rule preventive clinics of all types disregard financial status if persons make their first visit, come for purely educational services, or are referred by a private physician. Often diagnostic service is rendered to all who apply, as a satisfactory decision concerning further care can be reached only after the medical examination and recommendations for treatment have been made. If charges are made, they are nominal and are mainly for special procedures involving costs of material.

As so often happened in the history of health service, private initiative organized the first preventive clinics, and voluntary organizations, by experimentation and demonstration, convinced public opinion of the soundness and general applicability of the new idea. Once the way was paved governmental agencies began to share with nonofficial organizations in the further development of certain types of preventive services and in the extension of the movement to geographic areas not reached before.

In the United States the trend toward public responsibility for establishment of preventive clinics has been very distinct in recent years. The growth of such facilities has been rapid although highly uneven. Before the war governmental clinics were relatively dominant in some fields but uncommon—if not rare—in other fields of health activities. In general the large majority of services organized outside of hospitals and most of those in counties with less than 100,000 population were maintained by public agencies. Of the special services, most of those for preschool and school children and the majority of the immunization, dental, venereal disease, and tuberculosis clinics were government controlled. Responsibility for well-baby services was about equally divided between official and nonofficial agencies. A score of other activities, primarily maternal hygiene, birth control, orthopedic, eye, mental hygiene, and cancer clinics were mainly under the auspices of voluntary organizations.

The emergence of public responsibility for preventive health service in the United States is nothing unusual. Many foreign countries have committed themselves to a course clearly indicating their readiness to provide the implements of health protection. This general trend is well exemplified by the development that has taken place in the field of maternal and child health services in England and Wales. At the end of 1941, nearly four fifths of all clinics for infant welfare were maintained by local public agencies.

Significantly, the policy in determining the functions of government at various levels also follows a rather similar pattern. Establishment, operation, and administration of preventive clinics ordinarily is regarded as a local responsibility except where special conditions make this impracticable. Direction and equalization of the movement and standardization of service often have been accepted as a necessary function of the state or national government.

In the United States, Federal-state and state-local cooperation has been developed on a large scale since the adoption of the Social Security Act of 1935. This law with its amendment of 1939 provided for appropriations of Federal funds "for the purpose of assisting States, counties, and health districts and other political subdivisions of the States in the establishment and maintenance of adequate health services. . . ." A similar policy appeared in the Venereal Disease Control Act of 1938.

The principle of subsidizing local health facilities by the national government has been applied in a score of foreign countries. In many instances the allocation of grants-in-aid has been coupled with a requirement to provide for adequate clinic service. A few examples will serve to illustrate this point. The French law Léon Bourgeois of 1916 stipulated that national and local government jointly had to cover deficits of tuberculosis clinics. Moreover, it authorized the national government to make the establishment of such a service mandatory in any community which during five successive years had a tuberculosis mortality exceeding the national average. In Sweden (since 1918) and Norway (since 1923) legislation has been in effect which required larger communities to maintain public venereal disease clinics for both diagnosis and treatment. In Great Britain (since 1916) local authorities have been required to provide adequate facilities for treatment of venereal disease. They discharged this duty by steadily increasing the number of public treatment centers and making annual payments to nongovernmental clinics according to the amount of service rendered. The national government pays 75 per cent of the expenditures of local authorities.

PRIVATE GROUP CLINICS

The introduction of private group clinics was motivated by the desire of physicians to have a suitable basis for the development of group practice.

Group practice may be defined as a system of cooperative practice of medicine by physicians for the purpose of pooling experience and skill, facilities and equipment, technical and other auxiliary personnel, and operating expenses if not also earnings.[24] It aims at the improvement of quality, quantity, and effectiveness of medical care, the reduction of its costs, and the decommercialization of the practice of medicine. It constitutes an attempt to adjust medical practice to the rapid scientific progress and the profound socio-economic changes that have taken place since the nineteenth century.

A wealth of arguments have been advanced by the proponents of this new approach to the organization of medical service. They revolve about two major theses. In the first place, the rise of scientific medicine, with specialization as its characteristic feature, has greatly increased available knowledge and skill, scientific and technical. Medical care has become more efficient but also increasingly complex. To reap the full benefits that can be derived from this scientific advance and to make medical practice as effective as possible, the systematic association of the general practitioner with specialists and the close cooperation of the representatives of various medical specialties must be organized. Furthermore, the capital investment and operating costs necessary to conduct medical practice in accord with modern standards have been mounting steadily and constitute a heavy burden to the physician. From necessity, the price of good medical care has risen sharply. But the purchasing power of the average patient has not increased commensurately. The result is that a formidable economic barrier stands between those who are ready and willing to render service and those who want to obtain it. To effect economies and to pass them on to the patient, the cooperation of a number of physicians in the joint provision and utilization of the varied and expensive equipment, the technical and clerical personnel, and the physical plant is imperative.

Well-organized group practice conducted from a properly staffed and well-equipped center, such as a clinic or a hospital, would greatly benefit the patient, the health professions, and the community. It would provide for better and more service in a convenient way; serve to attain consistency and continuity of treatment; and reduce the costs of medical care for both patients and physicians. It would give the physicians and related groups opportunities for professional improvement through consultation, research, and postgraduate study; a satisfactory income; alternating freedom from night calls, Sunday work, and evening hours; and paid vacations. It would fill a gap in the community health program by making good medical care, both preventive and curative, available at reasonable costs.

Private group clinics for "the application of medical service by a number of physicians working in systematic association, with joint use of equipment and technical personnel and with centralized administrative and financial organization" [25] have been established more frequently since the first World War.

In the United States approximately four hundred private group clinics were believed to be in operation in 1942 as against about one hundred and fifty in 1930. Size and composition of the professional staffs vary greatly. There are very small groups with only three or four physicians working together. At the other extreme are organizations of more than eighty professional men, including physicians, dentists, and pharmacists. Groups of ten to twelve physicians are not uncommon, if only those are considered which are more than a family organization. In some instances general practitioners and partial specialists constitute the majority and full specialists the minority; in other instances the reverse is true. Most of the groups do not possess a hospital of their own. Patients needing hospitalization are referred to those institutions with which the individual physicians are affiliated or the group has made an agreement. The scope of service offered varies widely, ranging from diagnostic service only to a large variety of preventive and curative services at the clinic, the home of the patient, and the hospital.

The operation of a group clinic in itself does not necessarily imply a change in the traditional method of paying for service. In fact the vast majority of the private group clinics make use of the fee-for-service system, that is, patients are charged fixed fees according to the amount of service rendered. In some instances the principle of group practice has been combined with the principle of group prepayment. People who have joined a prepayment plan receive such care as is specified in the agreement without further payment and other services at preferential rates, while patients who are not subscribers have to pay the usual charges.

The income of the physicians ranges from about $3,000 for general practitioners in assistant positions to more than $10,000 for full specialists and medical directors. In general the scale allows for increases according to the number of years of service. These figures represent net income as all expenses for practicing medicine fall on the clinic budget. To the cash payments must be added the value of such common perquisites as paid vacations, paid time off to attend scientific meetings, allowances for short periods of postgraduate work, and liability and malpractice insurance.

THE CLINIC AND THE PHYSICIAN IN PRIVATE PRACTICE

The clinic movement in the United States has advanced without being part of a broad health program. The failure to organize physicians' services and to place the clinic in an integrated system of preventive services and care for the sick has caused an unending stream of controversies over the relationship between clinics and physicians in private practice.

The practicing physician who depends upon fees from patients for his livelihood must, by force of circumstances, insist that the clinic not interfere with private practice. Inevitably, any member of a health profession who has to struggle in competitive practice will closely scrutinize the clinic's work as to features carrying dangerous potentialities. The clinic in turn must respect the legitimate interests of the health professions. It has no choice but to draw some dividing line, artificial as it may be, between its areas of activity and the "territory" of the private physician.

The mere fact that clinics have increased in number and grown beyond their original function indicates that understandings between them and the health professions have been worked out locally. But it would be a self-deception to assume that more than a makeshift solution has been found. At present the prevention of "abuse of the clinic privilege" is the prime consideration determining the operation of clinics. Sincere efforts have been made to accomplish this end. Yet to some physicians the clinic has remained anathema and to others it is causing a sense of grievance easily fanned into flame by some unfortunate experience. Indicative of the restlessness in the medical profession is the following opinion published in the British medical journal *The Lancet:*

The growth of the public health services has subtracted much from his [the family doctor's] work. He has, speaking generally, no part in the antenatal services, the infant-welfare centers and the school medical services. This has not only seriously diminished his value and experience, but it has set up against him another group of doctors whose function is to supervise growth and nutrition, while he, for the most part, sees the family only in gross departures from health.[26]

It should not come as a surprise that the treatment clinics were the ones to be most frequently accused of encroaching on private practice. How old such complaints are and how early the clinic administrators tried to do their utmost to avoid friction with private physicians is illustrated by a report made in 1880. Dr. James H. Whittemore, discussing the subject "Are Free Dispensaries Abused?" had this to say:

In November, 1877, a competent and experienced man was employed [at the Massachusetts General Hospital Out-Patient Department] to investigate the condition of all who came to the department from Boston (old city) and South Boston. The result was as follows: number of visits, 386; number of deserving poor, 254; number giving wrong addresses, 79; number amply able to pay, 53. Of the fifty-three able to pay, nineteen owned their houses and other property in the city.

The statement was followed by a recommendation that there should be "a competent and experienced paid inspector at each of the large dispensaries" so as to prevent ineligible patients from receiving service.[27]

It testifies to the rigidity with which the private physicians' interests have been respected by treatment clinics that the percentage of abuse has been generally found to be small. A score of studies, many of them made under the auspices of medical societies, have shown that rarely over 4 and never over 10 per cent of the patients attending treatment clinics had to be classified as ineligible according to prevailing standards. The vast majority were found to be unable to pay for the same type and amount of service at private rates. Yet the argument never died, either in this country or abroad. Significantly, French physicians in 1936 resolved that *dispensaires* maintained by nonprofit voluntary organizations or public agencies should give only free treatment and exclusively to the indigent; and, in 1941, the Federal Council of the British Medical Association in Australia emphasized that out-patient departments should accept patients, except in an emergency, only if they produced "an introductory letter from their own practitioner."

While it was already hard enough to obtain some sort of agreement as to the manner of operating preventive services and the treatment clinics for the needy, it was even more difficult to arrive at an understanding on the function of group clinics for self-supporting people.

The principle of group practice has been applied not only by physicians in private practice but by a variety of organizations taking responsibility for the development of a nonprofit program of medical care. In the United States group clinics have been set up by industrial corporations, institutions of higher learning, consumer cooperatives, unions, and governmental agencies. In foreign countries, such as France, Germany, Chile, and Peru, they have been established under various auspices to serve patients covered by social insurance against sickness.

The appearance of group clinics was greeted by the medical profession with mixed feelings. On the one hand, their potential value to the improvement and extension of medical care was realized. On the other hand, their impact on the practitioner in individual practice was dreaded. How could the physician working in a solitary office compete, scientifically and economically, with a team of men pooling their skill and practicing under the most favorable conditions?

The first problem, then, was to decide whether group practice as such was "ethical" according to the rules governing professional conduct, and if so, what conditions of operations ought to be observed so as to avoid a violation of the principles of medical ethics.

In the United States the Judicial Council of the American Medical Association in 1932 made the following general statement: "A fundamental of medical ethics is that anything which in fact is opposed to the ultimate good of the people at large is against sound public policy and therefore unethical." The specific problem of group practice was commented upon by the Bureau of Medical Economics in its report to the House of Delegates of the American Medical Association for the year 1940 as follows:

Although the American Medical Association and its constituent societies have been charged with opposition to group practice, a search of the Proceedings of the House of Delegates of the American Medical Association for thirty-two years failed to show any action that indicated the slightest hostility to the formation of ethical and capable medical groups. The exent of the participation of group members as officials of the national and state organizations would indicate a complete absence of any such hostility.[28]

Opposition to unethical and incapable groups must be wholeheartedly supported by everybody genuinely interested in the improvement of medical care. However, there remains a delicate question. When is group practice unethical? Profound disagreement over this point has resulted in bitter controversies between the proponents of group practice and medical societies. The dispute arose when the physicians on the staff of a group clinic made an agreement with a third party to accept payment for their services on a basis other than the traditional fee-for-service system. In an effort to cover such cases the American Medical Association in 1934 amended its *Principles of Medical Ethics* by a section on "contract practice" as follows:

Contract practice *per se* is not unethical. However, certain features or conditions if present make a contract unethical, among which are: 1.

When there is solicitation of patients, directly or indirectly. 2. When there is underbidding to secure the contract. 3. When the compensation is inadequate to assure good medical service. 4. When there is interference with reasonable competition in a community. 5. When free choice of a physician is prevented. 6. When the conditions of employment make it impossible to render adequate service to the patients. 7. When the contract because of any of its provisions or practical results is contrary to sound public policy. . . .

The decision as to its [contract practice] ethical or unethical nature must be based on the ultimate effect for good or ill on the people as a whole.[29]

It is interesting to note that the French medical organization in 1936 set forth that *dispensaires mutuels* should be allowed to render service only to members of a mutual organization. Clinics for pay patients should be regarded as a commercial undertaking and frowned upon but tolerated if they were licensed as medical offices and made charges at least equal to the medical association's minimum fee schedule.

The long-standing controversy reached a climax in 1938 when the United States Department of Justice obtained the indictment of the American Medical Association on the grounds that it had restrained the lawful practice of medicine by restricting the activities of the Group Health Association of Washington, D.C. The case came before the Supreme Court, which in 1943, by unanimous ruling, upheld the conviction of the American Medical Association by the lower courts. The decision pointed out:

The medical societies combined and conspired to prevent the successful operation of Group Health's plan, and the steps by which this was to be effectuated were as follows: (1) to impose restraints on physicians affiliated with Group Health by threat of expulsion or actual expulsion from the societies; (2) to deny them the essential professional contacts with other physicians, and (3) to use the coercive power of the societies to deprive them of hospital facilities for their patients.[30]

UNSOLVED PROBLEMS

The very growth of the clinic movement has accentuated the need for a wise decision as to its future direction.

Should preventive and treatment clinics be merged, or should they be continued as functionally and administratively separated services?

Should clinics be organized for community use, or should they be maintained, as in the past, for the benefit of selected socio-economic groups?

Should medical centers be developed systematically in order to attain quality, efficiency, convenience, and economy of service through group practice?

These are complex questions. To answer them the crux of the problem must be considered. If the clinic is regarded as an appendage of medical practice, no change in the basic pattern of public policy is feasible. If the clinic is conceived as the center of both preventive health activities and medical care for the community, if it serves as the headquarters of physicians and related groups in private practice as well as of personnel employed by public and private agencies, reorientation of public policy is possible.

The fundamental issue, then, is whether medical practice should and can be organized on the basis of medical centers or whether such approach would be contrary to the best interests of the people to be served, the health professions, the hospitals, and the community.

· 4 ·

THE DEVELOPMENT OF PROGRAMS OF PUBLIC MEDICAL CARE FOR "PERSONS IN NEED"

IT IS simple to state that we want complete medical care of the finest type for the greatest number of people at the least expense. But it is a Herculean task to translate such theory into a practical and workable plan. Who shall have the right to obtain service at the expense of the taxpayer? This is one of the most vexatious problems with which public agencies have been struggling ever since taxes have been levied to defray costs of medical care.

THE GROUPS ELIGIBLE FOR PUBLIC MEDICAL CARE

In the United States public medical care is available to a considerable variety of selected groups of persons forming a sociological unit or living under similar economic conditions.

Apart from the members of the armed forces numerous groups of individuals are beneficiaries of provisions made by the Federal government. Among them veterans, merchant seamen, Indians and Eskimos, and certain groups of persons in the service of Federal agencies stand out as numerically strong. They all are in a class by themselves. With minor exceptions they are self-supporting; they are entitled to obtain all the care they need and are automatically eligible for service if they belong to one of the groups.

In an entirely different category of beneficiaries must be classified another, comparatively much larger, group of persons: namely, those financially unable to afford private care. They represent a group with small or no resources of their own and may be provided with some or all services on submitting an application. In any individual case, they must satisfy a considerable and widely varying number of eligibility requirements, including an investigation into the financial conditions of the family, to prove their need. The general policy and administrative procedure adopted in organizing medical care for such persons are of particular importance from the point of view of community health organization. They show the workings, potentialities, and relative merits of the public assistance approach to social security and, therefore, will receive primary consideration in the following presentation.

FROM THE "PAUPERS" TO THE "MEDICALLY NEEDY"

Public responsibility for persons who due to illness have lost or never possessed the capacity to function as productive members of their own community dates back to colonial times. It has found expression in the adoption of statutes modeled after the Elizabethan Poor Law Act of 1601. In principle, communities were ready to care for their most disadvantaged fellow citizens. In practice, they were unwilling to exercise this function in a way appropriate to the needs of a sick human being. For a long time the primary objective of public policy was, with the least expense, to dispose of a burden regarded as inevitable. Was it not true, as it says in Matthew 26, 11: "For ye have the poor always with you"? Was it not equally true that people had to be discouraged from becoming destitute lest self-supporting people would be penalized and taxpayers' money squandered? "Every penny bestowed that tends to render the condition of the pauper more eligible than that of the independent labourer is a bounty on indolence and vice." Such was the social philosophy enunciated by Lord Grey's Commission in England in 1832.[1] It was shared in many countries.

Repressing and deterring—this was the approach which seemed logical and natural in dealing with the poor, whether they were sick or not. Medical care at public expense was not denied. But it was restricted to a section of the population characterized solely by the fact that they had become destitute, and it was commonly given at the discretion of a lay "overseer of the poor." The early colonial statutes either referred generally to the relief of the "poor, old, blind, impotent, and lame persons, or other persons not able to work" with the inference that the sick were to receive care or they stated explicitly that provisions had to be made for "all the poor, lame, blind, sick and other inhabitants who are not able to maintain themselves." The sick who were "public charges" were classed with loafers, vagrants, beggars, and drunkards not only in the same statutes but also in the same institutions. Here and there a distinction was made which continued to be observed until the present: The "worthy" or "deserving" poor were accorded preferential status. Moralistic concepts frequently dominated both policy and procedure. Families were accepted for public medical care only if a thorough investigation had failed to produce any evidence of what was supposed to be a sin.

Formal application; the "means test," implying "inquiry into the state and circumstances of the applicant"; "the pauper's oath"; publication of the names of paupers; disfranchisement of civic rights; requirement to "work off" the costs of care; compulsion of relatives with "sufficient ability" to assume responsibility—all these practices were applied in the United States and in other countries alike, as though they were recommended by an international convention. They served effectively to keep the number of applicants for, and recipients of, public medical care at the irreducible minimum. Local communities tried to avoid expenses by confining service to citizens who could meet stiff residence and settlement requirements. Persons who were unfortunate enough to become sick before they had an opportunity to procure proper qualifications often were, at the earliest possible moment, removed to the place of their legal residence—if they had been able to acquire any; in some instances they were declared "State paupers." The states, in turn, tried to isolate themselves from difficulties common to all of them by barring nonresidents from the privilege of obtaining service. Although since the beginning of the nineteenth century a tendency developed to make special provision for a sick person not coming within the definition of a pauper, the conditions under which care could be obtained remained essentially unchanged.

Small wonder that application for public medical care came to be regarded as the last resort—to be shunned by any self-respecting citizen.

As the philosophy of repression of pauperism gave way to that of toleration, the divorce of public medical care from the worst features of the poor law became a much debated issue. The idea was advanced that "medical relief" should be treated differently from other forms of relief and not involve the recipient's being placed on the list of paupers. In the English-speaking world it was Ireland which made the first step in this direction. The Medical Relief Charities Act of Ireland, passed in 1851, declared that any poor person who was sick, although not necessarily a pauper, had the right to free advice and medicine and such was not deemed to be poor relief. About twenty years later an English committee recommended a similar policy. But public opinion in England was not yet ready to support such change. Too deep-rooted was the conviction that "people must not be encouraged to be ill by the knowledge that they could be treated free at the expense of the State." [2]

The broad policies and administrative practices adopted by a predominantly agricultural society for the relief of its sick "destitute or necessitous persons" enjoyed an exemplary longevity. In many countries they persisted well into the twentieth century despite the profound socio-economic changes brought about by the advent of industrialism. In some countries they still survive.

In 1526, a social seer, Juan-Luis Vivès, addressed a statement "Concerning the Relief of the Poor; or Concerning Human Need" to the Senate of Bruges urging the authority to do "what befits the state and the ruler thereof." He based his proposals on the following reasoning:

For those who care only for the rich and despise the poor, act just like a physician who should not think it of much importance to heal the hands or the feet because they are at a distance from the heart; but even as this would cause serious harm and suffering to the whole man, so also in the commonwealth the weaker may not be neglected without peril to the more powerful; for the former, driven by necessity, sometimes steal.[3]

It took society a long time to discover the fundamental truths that "the more powerful" could not be secure if a substantial fraction of the population was in want and that illness played a major role both as cause and result of want.

The number of persons depending upon public support began to increase. To paraphrase Mark Twain, there were many who due to illness were "fast rising from affluence to poverty." Lengthening relief rolls and mounting expenditures for the maintenance of the poor caused growing concern. A considerable number of individuals remained indefinitely on relief because little was done to remove the cause of their dependency, an illness or a defect amenable to medical treatment. Penny-wise official agencies sadly disregarded the long-term economic savings that could be achieved by providing for medical care to cure or improve a remediable condition and restore a relief client to at least some degree of employability, if not to full earning capacity and self-support.

"We want tax-paying citizens, not tax-eating citizens." This statement could be heard not infrequently but it remained one of aspirations. Public agencies were slow to admit that the system of poor relief was weak and self-defeating. When, in 1906, a British royal commission submitted a report on the Poor Laws, a minority had the wisdom and courage to make the following statement: "We accept responsibility for recommending the adoption of a Public Health principle of searching out disease in its incipient stages in place of the Poor Law attitude of waiting until the disease has gone so far as, on the one hand, to produce destitution, and on the other, to render the belated but costly treatment of no avail." But the time was not yet ripe for such a recommendation to be officially accepted.

The history of community health organization shows that it requires a great disaster to convince both peoples and governments of the inadequacy of health policies carried over from old times. Severe economic crises, rocking the foundations of national life in numerous countries, furnished the most potent arguments that ever swayed men's minds. It was mass unemployment and economic distress on a vast scale, multiplying the number and proportion of persons unable to support themselves, that forced Germany and Great Britain in the twenties and the United States in the thirties to substitute an entirely new system of public assistance for the outworn relief provisions. The Verordnung über die Fürsorgepflicht, adopted by the German Republic in 1924, the British Local Government Act of 1929 and Public Health Act of 1936, and the United States Social Security Act, passed in 1935, are typical examples of a general trend toward reorientation and expansion of public responsibility for social welfare. All these measures are nation-wide in scope. They are alike in embodying a constructive point of view instead of the negativistic attitude expressed in relief legislation. They put the dignity of the individual above his economic value; place major emphasis on the provision of "a reasonable subsistence compatible with decency and health" for those who have to depend upon public aid; and, by alleviating individual distress, try to prevent the cumulative effect of income deficiency upon individuals, communities, and the nation. They differ a good deal in details, though. Of general interest are some of the principles adopted abroad.

The German statutes differentiate among several groups of needy persons who are accorded a preferential status (*gehobene Fürsorge*) over the indigent in the old sense (*allgemeine Fürsorge*); stipulate that benefits and services be provided according to individual need; declare explicitly that medical care is an essential of life and must be made available as needed; and set as the ultimate aim of public assistance to make itself superfluous. The British statutes are noteworthy in various respects. They abandon the philosophy and practices of the Poor Laws in general. The new spirit is expressed in the simple but momentous sentence: ". . . all assistance which can lawfully be provided otherwise than by way of poor relief shall be so provided." To put the operation of public assistance on a firm basis an entirely new administrative organization is created. What is even more important, the whole system of public medical care is reorganized.[4]

The policy adopted in the United States rests on the tenet of "doing different things for different persons." Three groups of "needy" individuals are differentiated as meriting especial care: the old, dependent children, and the blind. For them special types of public assistance programs are operated on the basis of financial cooperation between the Federal government and the states.[5] The number of beneficiaries of these provisions necessarily fluctuates a good deal, not only from year to year but from month to month. In the continental United States in December, 1941, approximately 2,234,000 persons were receiving old-age assistance, 941,000 children (390,000 families) aid to dependent children, and 77,000 persons aid to the blind.[6]

Medical care is not mentioned in the sections of the Federal law referring to the three groups. However, it is made available to a considerable and steadily growing extent. To help beneficiaries of special assistance programs in paying bills for home visits, office care, and drugs or appliances, either special allowances are regularly included in their monthly cash benefits or additional payments are made if obligations are to be met. Significantly, more and more states have come to raise or remove the usual limit upon cash payments if medical care is needed.

That the policy of disbursing cash to the beneficiary is not conducive to the organization of good medical care has been generally recognized. Action to remedy the situation has been taken only in a small number of states. The state of Washington has distinguished itself by its determined efforts to provide for the old on a uniform state-wide basis. The Senior Citizens Grants Act, passed in 1941, established the right of persons at least sixty-five years of age to obtain more or less complete medical care at public expense.

With the development of special assistance programs for three preferred groups the problem of other needy persons was thrown into bold relief. The residual group that had to rely on general relief was not only large but had to be supported by the states and localities without financial aid from the Federal government. In the continental United States in December, 1941, there were approximately 798,000 cases receiving general relief. In addition, some 1,800,000 persons were employed under Federal work programs of various types.[7] They all depended upon public funds to meet their needs arising out of illness.

Since about 1930 medical care has been recognized as an "essential relief need." The establishment of the Federal Emergency Relief Administration program signalized the nation-wide acceptance of this principle. The right to obtain medical care at public expense has been incorporated in the public welfare statutes of many localities and a few states. There is, however, a great disparity in the provisions actually made for persons eligible for general relief. While selected services are provided in all sections of the country, fairly inclusive and well-organized programs are operated only in less than one fourth of all states.

It is hard to visualize a society without a certain proportion of persons needing public support so as to obtain the essentials of life, including medical care. But the problem must be seen in proper perspective. The fundamental issue at stake is to help as many people as possible not to become dependent because of serious illness or defect rather than providing for them only after they have exhausted their last resources and lost their economic independence.

Until recently public policy in the United States ignored the needs of sick people able to support themselves while in health. Nothing was done to attack the one source of poverty least difficult to dry up, sickness among people living on a precarious existence level. Little attention was paid to the obvious fact that the postulate "sink or swim" shelved but did not solve the problem of the sick—an experience painfully evident particularly to families with low income. Relief rolls were allowed to swell. Communities assumed responsibility for a debit yet were derelict in failing to conserve an asset. Efforts to reduce both frequency and duration of dependency caused by illness were sporadic and rare. The sick, the taxpayer, and society at large were the losers.

Persons who were not eligible for service at public expense and unable to pay the full costs of medical care found themselves in a serious dilemma. Should they deprive themselves of other necessities of life, pile up debts, or sacrifice assets badly needed for subsistence? Should they rely on the generosity of physicians in private practice or approach civic organizations or private welfare agencies for help? Should they apply for a "free bed" in a nongovernmental hospital, or attend one of the few treatment clinics operated by voluntary agencies for the benefit of people with small means? All these alternatives were used extensively. But they did not solve the problem. Self-supporting persons with low income often were worse off than recipients of public assistance. Moreover, the health professions and nongovernmental hospitals found it increasingly difficult to continue the noble tradition of giving their services free to those in need. In a spirit of resignation the low-income families, the health professions, and the voluntary hospitals tried to cooperate with the inevitable.

There is abundant evidence that the problem of "the forgotten man" has remained a live issue, much as it had been in 1883 when William Graham Sumner made his plea for "the simple, honest laborer, ready to earn his living by productive work" yet passed by "because he is independent, self-supporting, and asks no favors."[8] The specific problem of medical care that has arisen for self-supporting persons in general and those with low incomes in particular has been substantiated and clarified as to its nature and extent by a great body of painstakingly collected information on illness in relation to its social and economic setting.[9] Due to the change from an agricultural to a predominantly industrial economy about two thirds of the total national income before the war came from wages and salaries. Yet, in 1939, the median family income from these sources was only $1,231. On the other hand, the costs of good medical care have been mounting constantly, and more rapidly than the purchasing power of a large fraction of the population. The result has been a growing discrepancy between the standards for adequate medical care as set by experts and the quality and quantity of service actually received by all but a small proportion of the people.

Opinions clashed about the methods by which the general problem could best be solved. But there was wide agreement about a specific task that required immediate solution: the provision of medical care for people in the marginal income group where the disparity between need and services was most marked. The only way to accomplish this without a fundamental change in the traditional method of paying for medical care appeared to be the extension of service at public expense to the "medically needy."

Reinterpretation of concepts on public responsibility for persons who cannot provide for good medical care through their own resources has been urged time and again by a great many individuals and organizations. The medical profession, through representative bodies, has repeatedly stressed the need for adjustments to keep pace with newer developments.

The Committee of Physicians for the Improvement of Medical Care in 1937 stated "that an immediate problem is provision of adequate medical care for the medically indigent, the cost to be met from public funds (local and/or state and/or federal)"; in 1938 it reiterated that "the provision of adequate medical care for those who are unable to provide it for themselves is a public responsibility." [10] In 1938 the House of Delegates of the American Medical Association adopted a committee report declaring that "the medical profession as a whole will welcome the appropriation of [public] funds to provide medical care for the medically needy." [11] The "Platform" of the American Medical Association, offered in 1938, contained a recommendation for "the extension of medical care for the indigent and the medically indigent." [12]

Adoption of reasonable statutes is one of the prerequisites for the development of an adequate program of public medical care for persons unable to pay. Laws embodying modern concepts of social welfare and incorporating the principle of individual need rather than destitution as basis of social action have been passed in a few states only.

The Social Welfare Law of New York State, as revised in 1941, makes the public welfare district "responsible for providing necessary medical care for all persons under its care, and for such person[s], otherwise able to maintain themselves, who are unable to secure necessary medical care. The determination as to medical care necessary for any person shall be made with the advice of a physician." [13]

The Rhode Island General Public Assistance Act of 1942 makes eligible for aid all "persons in need in the state," regardless of citizenship, residence or settlement, and availability of small resources. General public assistance "may include necessary medical care and supplies and hospitalization." There are no restrictions on the granting of general public assistance "to needy persons who are unemployable" or "as supplementary aid, where needed, to persons receiving other types of assistance." Any local community is free to assist "out of local general relief funds, any person deemed eligible for assistance by a city or town who is not eligible in accordance with state standards." [14]

These two laws are noteworthy for their determined effort to liberalize the broad policies governing public medical care. Two other recent measures indicate a similar trend. It must be noted, however, that both apply to special conditions only rather than to illness in general. A Massachusetts law, passed in 1937, declares that sums paid by any town for the care of a prematurely born infant "shall not be deemed to have been paid as public relief, and no person shall be deemed to be in receipt of public relief because of his inability to pay such sums, but while such care is being given, such parent or person shall not acquire or lose or be in the process of acquiring or losing a settlement." [15]

Since early in 1943 special Federal funds have been allotted to the states to finance "emergency maternity and infant care" for wives and infants of enlisted men of specific grades in the armed forces.[16] Public medical care is made available on application without a means test, investigation, or a residence requirement. The economic base for eligibility is broadened. Care is provided when similar services are not otherwise readily available to the patient.

In the large majority of the states, however, the provision of public medical care is still governed by statutes containing unadulterated principles of the seventeenth century poor laws. Frequently a person in need, defined as a person who has no available real or personal property, is required to declare his "indigency and destitution," sign and swear to a statement to this effect, and file an application for aid in proper form before he can obtain some service. Even communities which make no distinction between the indigent in the legal sense and medically needy persons sometimes require a patient applying for medical care at public expense to sign a declaration like the following:

I, the undersigned, realize that the treatment and medicine provided free . . . is for those who cannot possibly pay for same, and hereby swear, that my condition is such that I must seek relief.

Within the limits drawn by statutes and available funds a number of communities have tried their best to improve the conditions under which public medical care can be obtained. A tendency has become manifest to avoid the application of the usual assistance standards if medical care is needed by a client. In some instances the eligibility levels for sick persons have been set considerably higher than for other persons in need. In other instances emphasis has been placed upon a strictly individualizing approach giving consideration to both the medical need and the socio-economic situation. Inevitably, there have come to the fore many intricate problems, such as the definition of medical need in general and the proper procedures in determining eligibility for public medical care in the particular case.[17]

Who is "medically needy"? This question has been raised ever since attempts have been made to proceed from the stage of a beautiful theory to the formulation of sound administrative practices. The definitions contained in the following two statements will serve to show what points representative organizations regard as important.

The American Medical Association in 1938 accepted a report by Dr. H. A. Luce stating:

A person is medically indigent when he is unable, in the place in which he resides, through his own resources, to provide himself and his dependents with proper medical, dental, nursing, hospital, pharmaceutical and therapeutic appliance care without depriving himself or his dependents of necessary food, clothing, shelter and similar necessities of life, as determined by the local authority charged with the duty of dispensing relief for the medically indigent.[18]

The American Hospital Association in 1942 adopted proposals on hospital care for the American people which included a recommendation for "the encouragement of local government payments to hospitals for service to 'needy' persons whose individual or combined payments are less than the costs of necessary service." [19]

Evaluation of the medical need of the individual in relation to his or his family's economic conditions, as recommended by these organizations, requires the adoption of norms rather than fixed rules in measuring need and of a flexible plan in providing service according to special conditions. Such steps have been taken by a number of communities. The standard budgetary requirements for the essentials of life and the probable costs, present and future, of the service needed are estimated and compared with the family's resources. The actual or potential "budgetary deficiency" is used to determine the extent to which medical care is provided wholly or partly at public expense.

In reorganizing their administrative practices many communities have followed the principles recommended in 1939 by the American Public Welfare Association:

Persons already accepted for maintenance at public expense should be accepted, without further investigation, for medical care at public expense.

The determination of medical need should be a medical responsibility and should precede the determination of financial eligibility.

Determination of eligibility should not delay necessary treatment.

Policies concerning determination of eligibility should be made by the public authority after consultation with the agencies and professions concerned; and should include agreement between agencies to avoid duplication of investigation.[20]

The principles of action recently applied to the organization of general programs of public medical care are not novel. On a selective basis persons other than recipients of relief have long been accepted for service at public expense. To support the effective campaign against certain diseases of social and economic importance, public medical care has been provided without considering destitution the criterion of eligibility.

Contagious diseases were the first to be singled out as requiring and warranting special measures. In the second half of the nineteenth century Great Britain relaxed the statutes governing public medical care by allowing for the hospitalization "of any person who is not a pauper suffering from any dangerous infectious disorder." The United States followed a similar course. The dominant influence shaping public policy was the desire to prevent danger to the community rather than to meet individual needs. As scientific progress offered new possibilities, communities began to organize treatment services to render infectious patients noninfectious and, thereby, reduce the frequency of infection. The conviction gained ground that the campaign against communicable diseases could be conducted effectively only if the broad policies and administrative procedures governing eligibility for medical care were entirely divorced from those observed in general. This led to the adoption of liberal standards in accepting patients with communicable diseases for care at public expense and to functional and administrative separation of services for the protection of the public health from others. One by one the old barriers set up against people unable to pay for treatment were let down. Poor-law principles were discarded, though not completely nor uniformly.

This trend is well exemplified by the development of public medical care for the more effective control of venereal diseases. In years of relatively normal incidence of communicable disease the reported cases of syphilis and gonorrhea led the list of all notifiable diseases in the United States. Their frequency, their impact on the individual and family life, and their socio-economic importance to the nation have brought about a movement to eliminate one of the most formidable obstacles to adequate treatment, namely the prohibitive costs. Following efforts on a small scale, a nation-wide program, aided by the allocation of Federal funds to the states, was inaugurated in 1938.[21] It rests on three major tenets: free diagnostic and treatment facilities for specified groups of people; free distribution of anti-syphilitic drugs on the request of any physician for the treatment of his patients; and availability of service irrespective of the place of residence of an infected patient. Public clinics have been established in large numbers. They accept all persons who apply for diagnosis and emergency treatment; those referred by a private physician for consultation or continued treatment; and those unable to afford private medical care.

That a well-organized and comprehensive system of public medical care is fundamental to the reduction of venereal diseases has long been recognized in many foreign countries. In particular, the Scandinavian countries, Germany, Russia, and—to a lesser degree—Great Britain have organized nation-wide programs that include tax-supported treatment services available to anybody who wants to use them, regardless of economic status.

Beside patients with communicable diseases, those with physical handicaps receive special attention in the United States. A typical example of early legislation embodying liberal eligibility standards in such cases is afforded by acts passed in Michigan in 1913 and 1915. They provided service at public expense for people who, though not in need of other relief, could not afford to pay for care. A nation-wide program of medical care for crippled children was developed through special provisions in the Social Security Act of 1935 and its amendments and rapidly extended by means of Federal-state cooperation. As a rule, the parents' financial ability to bear the cost of the treatment and care required rather than eligibility for public assistance has become the yardstick to measure qualification for obtaining service entirely or partly at public expense. The vast majority of the children cared for are in self-supporting families who could not readily meet the cost of specialists' services, extensive hospital care, appliances, and aftercare. Similar principles are embodied in the 1943 amendments to the Vocational Rehabilitation Act providing medical care for disabled civilian adults through a Federal-state program.

In assuming responsibility for persons unable to pay for medical care communities have come a long way. But there is still a long way to go.

It has become an established public policy to make certain provisions for recipients of public assistance in contrast to earlier times when only the poorest of the poor were considered "proper objects of public charity." There has been a growing tendency to meet the medical needs of persons with low income. As compared with some decades ago, not to mention earlier periods, a much larger number of those living on a precarious subsistence level—and a greater proportion of the population at that—now have the opportunity to obtain medical care at public expense.

In 1937 the American Public Welfare Association inquired into the policies of fifty large counties and cities. The "medically indigent" were excluded from public medical care in eight instances; they were eligible for any type of service in twenty-seven instances and for hospital care and for out-patient department treatment in ten instances, provided that their need had been established by investigation into their financial condition. In addition, special types of cases or categories, such as "emergencies" and Work Progress Administration employees were included in five instances.[22] In advanced communities "cases opened for medical care only" have numerically and proportionately increased up to the end of 1941. However, communities restricting service to recipients of special assistance and general relief greatly outnumber those fostering liberal policies. Moreover, many of the public agencies theoretically ready to aid marginal-income families have set their eligibility standards so low that little room is left for service to persons other than those in gravest emergencies or dangerously close to the relief level. Such patients who are not poor enough to qualify for public medical care are left to the charity of private organizations, voluntary hospitals, and health professions, if not to the mercy of loan sharks.

In some parts of the country determined efforts have been made to purify the atmosphere of the poor-law, so offensive to applicants for medical care. On the whole, progress has been slow. Residence and settlement requirements, inadequate eligibility standards, legal family responsibility, administrative practices subjecting applicants to indignity, and local responsibility for care have continued to dominate the scene and retard the development of adequate programs of public medical care.

Serious as these shortcomings are, they can be removed by adjusting both broad policies and administrative practices to the needs of today. But there looms a larger problem. Application for aid and establishment of eligibility, determined on the basis of a means test including an investigation into the financial condition of the family, are the prerequisites for service at public expense. Such requirements cannot possibly be abolished if the patient's inability to pay determines the beginning, scope, and end of action on the part of public agencies. Is it in the interest of the sick with small resources, the health professions, the hospitals, and the community to continue this policy?

FROM EMERGENCY SERVICE TO ORGANIZED PROGRAMS

The formulation of a medical care program which would be fair to the needy sick, the health professions, the institutional facilities, and the taxpayer requires realism as well as vision. The efficient and economical operation of such a plan depends not only on the establishment of sound administrative policies and procedures but also on the spirit in which the day-to-day work is performed. It ought to be the spirit of social service rather than that of relief.

Leaning on the experience accumulated in a number of progressive communities, the American Public Welfare Association has taken the initiative and leadership in advancing the organization and administration of adequate medical care for persons who cannot provide for it through their own resources. In 1939 this organization stated the "Essentials of Tax-Supported Medical Service" to be as follows:

1. Scope and amount of care sufficient to include all necessary preventive and curative service required by persons unable to procure it for themselves.
2. Good quality of service and of personal attention.
3. Reasonable accessibility and promptness of service.
4. Continuous care of the patient, including:
    a. Continuity of diagnosis and treatment by different types of service—home, ambulatory and hospital;
    b. Continuity of preventive and curative service;
    c. Integration of medical and social treatment.
5. Reasonable payment to all participating medical practitioners * and agencies.
6. Participation of medical professions * and agencies in planning service; and as wide a participation in furnishing service as is compatible with quality, scope and economy.
7. Economy of expenditure, consistent with adequate scope, amount and quality of service.
8. Provision of service under conditions which will encourage its full use; avoidance of conditions which will deter the needy from securing necessary medical care or discourage well-qualified practitioners or agencies from participating in the service.
9. Adequate records of professional service and expenditure.[23]

Such an outline raises intricate questions. Shall the plan provide for all or selected services? If limitations are believed unavoidable, which services shall be chosen for inclusion in the program? Shall access to the available services be unrestricted or subject to certain conditions? What is the best method of organizing and paying for the services of professional personnel and institutional facilities? What administrative organization shall be created to assure the smooth functioning of the plan and promote high standards of service?

The scope of an adequate program of medical care must be wide. Ambulatory, domiciliary, and institutional care; all necessary preventive, diagnostic, corrective, and curative services; and indispensable supplies must be available in an amount and for a period sufficient to meet the needs arising out of sickness, injury, and maternity.

A broad program must be well-balanced, with no duplications or gaps. Emphasis on one or a few essential services with neglect of others equally essential would seriously hinder the successful operation of the entire plan.

* "Physicians, dentists, nurses, medical social workers and pharmacists."

A program meeting these requirements holds great promises for the attainment of early diagnosis, early and effective treatment, completeness of care, and consistency and continuity of service. If it is well-organized and intelligently operated it serves to prevent needless suffering and anxiety, unnecessary expenditures, and waste of effort.

The types of care provided for persons in need now differ sharply from those made available in earlier times.

Originally, "outdoor relief" in the form of physicians' service at the office and in the home of the patient was granted. Soon public policy took an entirely different course. The main emphasis was placed upon provision of institutional care. Typical examples of this trend are afforded by developments in Detroit and in the state of Connecticut. At the beginning of the nineteenth century the city of Detroit provided for outdoor relief. Later it decided to abandon this type of care because its costs increased "beyond expectations." A poorhouse was opened in 1832.[24] Connecticut in 1886 added provisions for some medical care of "paupers" to the statutes but, at the same time, stipulated "all must be kept in an almshouse." [25]

The institutions of the poorhouse type served the sick along with the well. There, the "blind, old, lame, sick or decrepit" were huddled together and, inevitably, the sick, defective, and disabled congregated and increased appreciably. The abominable conditions prevailing in such institutions in Michigan in the early eighteen seventies have been vividly described by Isabel C. Bruce and Edith Eickhoff.[26] They were, however, not worse than elsewhere at that time.

In short, until the latter part of the last century there was little public medical care—and that was utterly inadequate. Yet the very agencies which conspicuously disregarded the needs of the sick—and thereby the welfare of the community—were willing and ready to act upon the death of an indigent person. Bills for "coffins for paupers" were accepted, and they were numerous and high. Statements concerning "medical treatment of town charges" were disputed; if approved they were paid at arbitrary and low rates. The theory of inexpensive government, thus, was carried to the point of absurdity.

With the development of the modern hospital public medical care entered a new phase. Hospitalization became the favorite form of "relief of the sick," although the use of almshouses was not discontinued. Clinic service was provided more frequently, primarily in large cities. Home care was not organized, although there were a few exceptions to the rule.

As hospital service improved, the seriously ill—in the South called the "powerful sick"—could and did receive the best care there was. In areas where clinics were operated, persons able to walk or travel short distances could obtain at least certain essential services and, in some instances, care of high quality. On the other hand, the number of treatment clinics was much too small, and provisions for care at the physician's office and in the home of the patient were much too uncommon to change the situation fundamentally. The patient had no opportunity to procure for himself the type of care best suited to his condition nor all the services needed. The physician, trying to live up to the noble tradition of his profession, had to carry a heavy burden in giving freely of his time, and often of his money, to attend the needy sick as best he could in their homes, in the hospital, and in his office. Public agencies experienced mounting expenditures for free hospital care. In the absence of other more economical provisions patients had to be hospitalized frequently and for relatively long periods.

The third phase of public medical care began with the inclusion of home and office care in the scope of provisions, the extension of clinic care, and the introduction of unified permanent programs designed to meet modern standards of adequacy.

Home care in cases of sickness and maternity—according to Michael M. Davis long "the stepchild of public medical services"—has been receiving more attention since the early nineteen thirties. Among the first states to accord this type of care official recognition was New York, which in December, 1931, released state-wide "Regulations Governing Medical Care in the Home to Recipients of Home Relief." The strongest impulse to a revision of public policy came from the Federal government which under the terms of the Federal Emergency Relief Administration Act of September, 1933, allotted funds to pay for home care. With the withdrawal of these grants at the end of 1935 many communities with meager financial resources were temporarily thrown back to the point at which they had been before. Others not only retained but built up home care and made it the basic form of "medical relief." In general, there developed a definite trend toward provision of this type of service.

By 1940 home visits of physicians were paid from general public assistance funds in about four fifths of all states and from other funds in a large number of jurisdictions. They were, however, not provided in all communities within these states.

Service at the physician's office also has been made available at public expense more frequently than in earlier times. It is now organized in the majority of states in a number of communities, and in a few states in nearly all localities.

In general, the identification of public medical care with institutional care has become a thing of the past. There are still communities in which an institution of the poorhouse type is the only facility available for the care of chronically sick, permanently disabled, and mentally disturbed persons without resources of their own. There are still a few states stipulating in their statutes that general relief funds can be used to pay for care in almshouses and poor farms only.[27]

Distinct, indeed, is the trend toward provision of ambulatory, domiciliary, and hospital care without discrimination. However, not only the broad policies but also the administrative practices vary greatly from state to state, from locality to locality within the same state, and even from agency to agency within the same community.

The types of service included in modern programs of public medical care are many and varied in contrast to some decades ago when they were few and undiversified. Progressive communities have come to recognize the necessity of services formerly considered luxuries and the economy of ample provisions formerly branded as extravagant.

The direction of public policy in extending and improving the services for persons in need is indicated in the following recent developments.

1. Certain specialists' services outside of hospitals and out-patient departments have been made available.

2. Consultants have been appointed by public agencies. Most of them are obstetricians, pediatricians, and orthopedists, while psychiatrists, ophthalmologists, and other specialists are employed relatively infrequently. Their duties include giving advice and assistance to practicing physicians with less specialized training and experience.

3. Dental treatment has been organized for certain groups, such as preschool children, school children, and adults on the basis of widely varying plans. Complete care is rare. Extractions are pro-

vided often, certain fillings not infrequently, and other preventive and restorative services rarely.

4. Bedside nursing in the home in cases of sickness, maternity, or both has been developed somewhat more frequently.

5. Medical social service has been included in the programs of a growing number of communities.

6. Diagnostic laboratory and roentgenological services have been greatly extended.

7. Drugs, medicines, and certain diets have been provided more liberally, particularly all the preparations needed for the treatment of venereal disease, pneumonia, and malaria.

8. Selected surgical and orthopedic appliances, and eyeglasses—including reading glasses in some instances—have been increasingly supplied at public expense.

9. Ambulance service to hospitals and transportation to clinics have been included in the provisions for the needy.

Most or all of the essential services have been made available to persons in need in approximately one fourth of the states through state-wide programs, and in a considerable number of communities on the basis of local plans. Hospitalization has been emphasized by the vast majority of communities, on the theory that only serious illness warrants public action. On the whole, the exclusions by far exceed the inclusions. Complete medical care is organized only for a small fraction of the needy population.

As a general rule, details as to scope of service are not specified by law. An exceptional policy has been adopted in the state of Washington. There the law stipulates that persons eligible for public medical care under the "Senior Citizens Grants Act" be provided with "medical, dental, surgical, optical, hospital and nursing care" and also "artificial limbs, eyes, hearing aids and other needed appliances." [28] According to administrative interpretation other items "such as false teeth, crutches and glasses" also are included.

In sharp contrast to the approach used in providing for those sick persons who are customarily classified as needy, public policy has emphasized the development of well-rounded plans of public medical care for the effective campaign against certain diseases and defects. Particularly noteworthy for their inclusiveness are the provisions for crippled children and for family dependents of enlisted men.

The crippled children's programs cover "services for locating crippled children, and for providing medical, surgical, corrective, and other services and care, and facilities for diagnosis, hospitalization, and after-care." In addition to medical care, educational and vocational services as well as social work are made available through separate programs. "The whole child, not just his crippling condition, is given consideration in the provision of adequate medical care. Many supplementary services, all interdependent and each indispensable, are integrated in a satisfactory program." [29]

Under the emergency program for wives and infants of enlisted men payment is made by the states for the following services: (1) medical services (and, when necessary, surgical services) provided by physicians for complete maternity care (a) throughout pregnancy, labor, and six weeks post partum, (b) for major intercurrent conditions occurring during but not attributable to pregnancy, and (c) for the care of sick infants; (2) consultant services of specialists; (3) hospital care for maternity patients and sick infants whenever needed and for whatever period of time necessary; (4) immunization of infants against smallpox, diphtheria, and whooping cough; (5) bedside nursing care for maternity patients and infants when requested by the attending physician; (6) other services such as blood for transfusions and ambulance service when requested by the attending physician.

In advanced communities the general programs for persons in need and the special programs for the control of certain diseases and defects, although conducted separately, complement each other functionally, contingent upon the efficiency of the administrative organization of health service. However, the very fact that there are vast differences in the scope of provisions depending upon such artificial demarcation as type of disease has served to accentuate the need for a complete revision of the broad policy in regard to public medical care.

Ready access to public medical care must be assured. There is no place in modern society for the inhumane, unrealistic, and uneconomical practices of earlier times which confined public medical care to patients in dire emergency or put so many limitations on the use of existing services that the restrictions approached the point of absurdity.

The broad objectives of social action in making public medical care readily available are undisputed. Early diagnosis and treatment must be encouraged. Good services must be delivered at the point of need; at the time of need; in an adequate amount; and over a sufficient period of time. Needless suffering as well as expenditures for the maintenance of sick, disabled, and unproductive persons must be reduced if not prevented.

The attainment of these objectives has been impeded by the difficulties that must be overcome in proceeding from the talking to the acting stage. Should public medical care be provided "if necessary" or on the basis of more detailed specifications? Actually, general statements allowing for wide latitude in interpretation have been preferred to narrow and necessarily unsatisfactory definitions. Some of the newer public assistance statutes contain the simple but consequential declaration that "necessary medical care" must or may be provided.

But here arises another question. What are the conditions that make service necessary? Should acute and chronic illness and diseases and defects be treated equally? Should "unemployable" and employable persons receive the same type, scope, and amount of service? The following statute and administrative rules answer some or all of these questions.

An act passed in Tennessee in 1939 declares "that the terms 'medical care' and 'medical service' . . . are intended to describe and define care or services rendered an individual for the relief of some disease or abnormality, and is intended to be distinguished from the services customarily rendered by Public Health Departments." [30]

The "Procedural Instructions" issued by the New York State Department of Social Welfare state: "The scope of the individual items listed in the Analytical Chart [of Reimbursable Care] includes necessary preventive, diagnostic, corrective and curative services, and supplies essential thereto, provided by qualified medical and related personnel for conditions in a person that cause acute suffering, endanger life, result in illness or infirmity, interfere with his capacity for normal activities, or threaten some significant handicap." [31]

The rules and regulations of the Chicago Relief Administration authorize service for acutely ill and chronically ill persons regardless of the probability of rehabilitation.[32]

The advance of concepts regarding types of care, types of service, and accessibility of public medical care for the needy is well exemplified by the development in New York State. There the locally admin-

PROGRAMS FOR "PERSONS IN NEED"

istered medical care plans now may provide for all forms of medical care including—regardless of the extent of State participation—many or all of the following:

Acute illness, home or office
Ambulance service
Boarding homes for invalids
Chronic illness, home, office, etc.
Clinic care, by referral
Consultant services
Dental care, including
    Prophylaxis
    Treatment
    Fillings
    Extractions
    Dental surgery
    Dentures
Drugs, sera, etc.
Eye examinations
Eyeglasses and glass eyes
Fractures
Hospital care
Laboratory services
Major surgery, home or hospital
Medical services in hospital
Minor surgery
Nursing care, including
    Visiting nurse, per visit
    Registered nurse, per day
    Practical nurse, per day
    Home medical aides
Nursing home care
Obstetrics; home or hospital
Physiotherapy
Pneumonia treatment
Preventive services, by referral
Prosthetic or surgical appliances
Radium treatment
Sickroom supplies
Specialist services
Tuberculosis treatment, home
Venereal disease treatment
X-ray diagnosis
X-ray treatment [33]

The Chicago Relief Administration has adopted a program of dental care under which a large variety of services may be authorized.

For children "preventive and restorative operative dentistry in all its branches" is made available with the exception that orthodontic procedures and the use of precious metals for filling materials are excluded.

Services for adults include: Operative dentistry for relief of pain and elimination of infection; root canal therapy in rare cases; prophylaxis under certain conditions with cleaning and polishing of teeth for purely aesthetic reasons being excluded; fillings (cement, amalgam, synthetic porcelain); repairs of dentures; surgery (simple extractions, removal of impacted teeth when necessary for relief of pain or protection of health, fractures of jaws); roentgenograms if imperative for diagnostic purposes; and, subject to special approval, major oral surgery in emergency cases, partial or complete dentures under certain conditions, bridgework in rare instances, and emergency dental service in the home for bed-ridden patients.[34]

PROFESSIONAL SERVICES: ORGANIZATION AND PAYMENT

The satisfactory organization of professional services for the needy in the home, office, clinic, hospital, and custodial institution caused a good deal of headache to both public agencies and health professions even at a time when public medical care was in its infancy and the needy were few. It has become a crucial issue ever since inclusive programs have been initiated for the large number of people unable to afford good medical care at private rates.

The basic questions that require a wise decision are two, and they are closely related: (1) What system of organizing professional services shall be adopted? (2) What method of paying for professional services shall be chosen? The way in which these problems are solved determines the quality, quantity, and cost of medical care obtainable to those depending upon public aid.

There is no dispute about the objective to be attained. Adequate professional service must be assured at the lowest cost consistent with high standards. This implies that the interests of the patients, the health professions, the taxpayers, and the community as a whole must receive due consideration. Can they be reconciled? No final answer to this question is on record. The search for the best method of organizing and paying for professional services has been protracted and intensive. It still continues. Many and diverse arrangements have been tried out in the course of centuries. Of the old practices, some have been widely abandoned because of their glaring defects. Others, although admittedly deficient, have been continued essentially as before, since local conditions have been unfavorable to change. Still others have been completely revised in the light of modern ideas. New methods have rarely been tested. The unholy alliance of indifference and parsimony that exerted such powerful influence on public policy in earlier times still rules in a goodly number of communities.

Physicians' Service [*]

In the early days there was but one thought in the minds of administrators of public medical care. Tax funds had to be conserved to the utmost. What was more natural—and at the same time more economical—than to rely on the generosity of the physician who

---

[*] The basic principles discussed in this section equally apply to the organization of dentists' service.

traditionally had given freely of his skill and time and money to help the poor? Typical of such reasoning is the action taken early in the nineteenth century by the Common Council of Detroit. For those persons "whose pecuniary circumstances render them objects of their benevolence," the "gratuitous services of the Medical Gentlemen of the City" were "respectfully solicited." [35]

Another saving device was used in Boston and, later, in other communities fortunate enough to become the seat of a school of medicine. The Overseers of the Poor of that town in 1810 voted to allow professors of Harvard College to visit the sick in the almshouse "for the purpose of remarking on the nature of cases" and teaching the students "the best methods of treatment and mode of care." Cool-calculating businessmen that they were, they stipulated that the sick "should receive . . . all necessary medical attention and medicine, free from expense to the Town." [36] Thus, both sides struck a bargain, and the sick in the almshouse were the winners.

Such practices had at least one advantage. They created a clear-cut situation. Not so with other policies increasingly favored and widely used by officials in charge of poor relief.

Professional services as well as boarding, nursing—and even burials—were "let out" to the lowest bidder on a flat rate basis. In Kern County, California, for instance, in 1877 a contract to "furnish medical and surgical attendance and all medicines and surgical supplies to all patients who might be hospitalized" was awarded to a physician bidding $116 per month.[37]

Experience soon furnished abundant evidence of the shocking defects inherent in such a system. There was no guarantee that the patients received the care needed. Fierce competition forced the bidding down to ridiculous levels. The physicians who waged the mercenary battle and those who captured the contract were not necessarily the most respected and competent professional men. At the end of the contract year, the unscrupulous doctor, doing as little as possible for the sick, could record a handsome profit, while the conscientious discovered a deficit. Inevitably many physicians became convinced that a fair deal could never be expected from a governmental agency.

These facts alone, one may be inclined to assume, should have induced public agencies once and for all to discard the practice of "renting the sick out." Yet, such is not the case. In some parts of the country the outworn method is still in use, and here and there it has even remained on the statute books.

Besides contracting for medical service official agencies not infrequently resorted to other practices. On application a special fee was voted for a special case or a small remuneration allowed for services rendered to a "public charge." Occasionally a lump sum was appropriated to pay doctors' bills or the physician whom the administrator thought would charge the least was given an "order." Haggling over the amount of payment developed frequently, involved a host of litigations, caused a great deal of lost motion of the administrative machinery, and created a feeling of deep bitterness among the physicians. Neither these practices nor the disputes have become entirely a thing of the past.

Communities with modern programs of public medical care employ a great variety of methods to make the services of physicians available in a systematic way. According to the basic principles of organization two systems may be distinguished. Both are old but have been greatly modified to meet modern requirements.

Under the first system all physicians in private practice in a certain area may be admitted to a plan for organized care of the needy sick if they so desire and accept the terms. Their names are entered on an official list, the "panel." This policy recognizes, within legal and economic limitations, the traditional relationship existing between the patient and the physician. Its aims are well expressed in the following statement: "The essential thing, we consider, is to bring the medical treatment of the sick poor into line with that of other classes, and to ensure that for as many persons as possible poverty will not interrupt continuity of medical supervision by the family doctor." [38]

In actual practice either all licensed physicians with offices in a certain area or only the members of the local medical society are eligible. Occasionally a "rotating panel" is organized so as to allow physicians to work part of the year alternately. The patient who qualifies for public medical care is free to choose his doctor from among those participating in the program. However, free choice often is limited to general practitioners while special arrangements are made to assure the services of specialists and consultants.

Under the second system a varying number of physicians are appointed or selected on a merit basis to serve part-time or full-time. The sick who want to obtain care at public expense and are found to be eligible must seek the services of these physicians.

Some communities use one system preferably or exclusively, others, both in combination. In many sections of the country it is settled policy to maintain clinics and require all ambulatory sick in need to obtain either specialists' or all services there.

A characteristic of the present situation is the great disparity in the methods locally employed to provide physicians' service at the home of the patient, the office, clinic, hospital, and custodial institution. For home and office care, the "free-choice panel system" and the "district physician system" are utilized widely. The city, county, or district physician, the modern counterpart of the parish and town doctor, usually is assigned to a geographic area or political unit to attend all the needy living in the district. In most of the communities he serves on a part-time and in some on a full-time basis. His duties are either limited to home care or extended to include office care and supply of ordinary drugs. In a few large cities full-time physicians attached to a public hospital or out-patient department attend the sick in the home.

In providing for clinic service the prevailing policy is to rely on the personnel resources available at the institution rather than to conclude specific agreements. Exceptions to this rule are made in communities operating unattached treatment clinics. In such cases, a certain number of physicians are regularly employed, usually for certain hours a week.

Medical service for patients in general hospitals is in the large majority of communities given by those physicians in local practice who have "hospital privileges" and infrequently by a closed staff of full-time men whose duties include the care of ward patients. County homes and similar institutions of the custodial type often have part-time and occasionally full-time physicians.

Since the early thirties a tendency has appeared to incorporate the free-choice principle in administrative rules and laws. There have been some precedents to such policy. The Indiana Poor Law of 1838, for example, stated that the poor should be attended by "such physicians . . . as the sick shall prefer." Under the Federal Emergency Relief Administration Act of 1933, which allocated Federal funds for home care, the principles were enunciated that, so far as possible, the opportunity to participate in the service should be open to all qualified practitioners, and that free choice of physician by the patient should prevail. Similar were the administrative practices later adopted by a number of local communities. A typical example is afforded by the Chicago Relief Administration's *Rules and Regulations Governing Physicians' Services*. They declare:

> Medical care shall be supplied, in so far as is possible, by the physician who has previously cared for the patient. Each patient shall be permitted to consult the physician of his choice. If he has no family physician, the patient shall be asked to choose from the three physicians whose names appear next on the rotating list of physicians whose offices are located within the boundaries of the district from which the patient receives relief.[39]

Laws recently passed in some states explicitly refer to the method of organizing physicians' services. In the state of Washington, according to the act of 1941, the sick eligible for old-age assistance must be provided with medical care "by a doctor of recipient's own choosing." [40] In the state of Minnesota an act adopted in 1939 stipulated that where state funds are utilized in providing relief "all recipients of public relief shall be permitted free choice of vendor for supplies and services, on written relief orders, provided that the vendor thus chosen shall conform to the regulations of the State and local relief agencies." [41]

In the state of Michigan a law of 1941 states:

> "The private physician-patient relationship shall be maintained . . ." but it adds: ". . . nothing in this section shall be construed as affecting the office of any city physician or city pharmacist established under any city charter or of any county health officer or of the medical superintendent of any county hospital." Finally the law says: ". . . eligible sick shall be permitted to select either a private professional attendant . . . or the city physician or city pharmacist established under any city charter." [42]

Finally the United States Congress, in 1943, in appropriating funds for obstetrical care of wives of enlisted men made the proviso that no patient should be prevented "from having the services of any practitioner of her own choice, paid for out of this fund, so long as State laws are complied with." [43]

Measures such as those enacted by the legislatures of Washington and Minnesota and by the Congress have raised rather than settled delicate questions. Shall free choice of "doctor," "vendor," or "practitioner" be construed as implying freedom of the patient to select the services of licensed nonmedical practitioners? Shall free choice of physician be interpreted as applying only to home and office care or also to clinic and hospital care? Shall it be restricted to general practitioners' services or extended to specialists' services? Does a community comply with the law if it offers the patient choice between panel and salaried physicians?

The methods of paying physicians other than those employed full-time are so diverse that only very broad statements can be made.

Physicians appointed on a part-time basis receive a fixed salary, usually per month, with or without allowances for transportation depending upon the type of their work. In rare instances, they are paid a flat fee per eligible person or per call.

Under the organized panel system public agencies and physicians conclude a more or less formal agreement as to the method of payment, the fees, and the administrative procedures for the control of expenditures, thus substituting collective bargaining for individual understandings. The principle of authorization of service is generally applied.

Where a fee-for-service system is chosen the physicians are compensated for medical attention and transportation in proportion to the amount of authorized work actually done and on the basis of a special fee schedule adapted to local conditions. As a rule the fees are set below those ordinarily charged in view of the fact that reimbursement is certain while collections in private practice usually represent only a certain proportion of the charges.

Often, the discount is graded according to the type of service performed. Some communities allow the participating physicians a flat rate according to the number of people eligible for service at a given time (capitation system) or the number of sickness cases actually attended, regardless of the amount of service given in the individual case.

Not infrequently a fixed amount of money per month or year is paid into a pool and distributed, or prorated if necessary, among the physicians in proportion to the service actually rendered.

Often, different methods of payment are used in combination. Agreed fees are paid to specialists for approved service and flat rates to general practitioners for the work covered by an agreement.

The prepayment method, long used by self-supporting persons, has recently been employed by a few public authorities to compensate physicians for service to designated groups. The official agency transfers to the local medical society a certain sum per case per month in advance; the physicians in turn furnish such services as are specified in the agreement. Such plans have been developed primarily in Kansas.[44]

It is quite common that a variety of payment methods are employed not only within the same state but also within the same county. The multiplicity and diversity of practices does not end with this, however. There are cities where different payment arrangements are made for service to different groups of needy persons.

An interesting example of newer trends is afforded by the development in Kansas. In 1942, of 105 counties with organized care of the needy, 84 had free-choice plans (panel system) and 21 had county physician plans. Payment under the panel system was made on the basis of lump-sum allocations in 5 instances, fee-schedules in 51 instances, and prepayments in 28 instances.[45]

While it is true that orderly arrangements for the payment of physicians are slowly taking the place of arbitrary and make-shift procedures, it is equally true that there are surprising inconsistencies in the policies of public agencies. Professional services in the home of the patient or at the office of the physician are now paid for in many communities, while work at the clinic or in the hospital very often is not. In 1936, of more than 20,000 physicians engaged weekly in out-patient department service, only 8 per cent received an honorarium.[46] In contrast those on the staff of unattached treatment clinics usually were paid. So were the many doctors serving at such tax-supported institutions as tuberculosis and venereal disease clinics or in charge of well-baby conferences and school health service. Physicians attending needy patients in general hospitals rarely are remunerated by public agencies. Traditionally, they have been expected to give their services free to ward patients without resources of their own on the theory that experience, prestige, and spiritual uplift constituted the return for charitable work. However, such reasoning has not been followed consistently. The special hospitals under government control usually employ salaried physicians for service to all patients regardless of economic considerations.

*Relative Merits of Various Methods of
Organization and Payment*

The community which considers the introduction of an adequate, economical, and efficient program of public medical care must carefully weigh the relative merits and feasibility of the various methods of organizing and paying for medical service. There is no such thing as a golden rule applicable everywhere. Nor are arrangements which have proved their value in some communities ready for immediate use elsewhere. However, there is a wealth of accumulated experience clearly indicating the advantages and disadvantages inherent in each of the principal systems of organization and payment.

The free-choice system makes it possible for the needy patients to obtain, without discrimination, the services of any of the physicians participating in the local program; to remain under the general care of the same doctor regardless of the vicissitudes of life; and to change the physician within certain geographic, time, or other limits. It relieves the sick from the strain of traveling to some distant point for service. Because of its competitive aspects, it promises ready response to calls and eagerness on the part of the physician to give his best. The doctor is offered an opportunity to render service to the needy and receive payment for it. He can establish new relationships with patients hitherto not seen at all or attended irregularly. He can reinforce the bond of sympathy and interest between himself and his old patients. To the public agency the free-choice system is attractive because it is certain of ready acceptance by the medical profession.

On the debit side of the ledger are numerous more or less unavoidable weaknesses in the free-choice system. Many patients choose and change the physician on conditions that have little or nothing to do with professional experience and skill.[47] They drift to the "busy doctor" recommended by a close associate, the neighbor, drug store clerk, barber or beautician, or to the one most ready to meet all their requests. Not all physicians in active practice in a locality care to participate in a program. Often the names of the best trained and most experienced practitioners, particularly specialists, are conspicuously missing on the official list of physicians available for home and office care. Yet these very physicians serve the needy in the hospital wards and clinics where there is no free choice. Time and again experience has shown that there is a tendency, especially in cities, for the bulk of home care "to fall into the hands of a relatively few of the less able practitioners." [48] Quality of care is hard to promote, if license to practice medicine rather than qualification to perform certain services is all that is required for admission to panel practice. High standards of service cannot be maintained unless the medical profession agrees to assume full responsibility for the guidance and supervision of the professional performance of its members, is determined to discharge such function resolutely, and is empowered to take all steps necessary to achieve the desired results.

The combination of the free-choice panel system with the fee-for-service method rather than the capitation system of payment multiplies and intensifies its shortcomings. To control the expenditures and prevent excessive use, if not abuse, of the service by both patients and physicians, a host of rules and regulations must be worked out and enforced. The patient has to obtain authorization to seek medical attention at public expense. This may involve several money- and time-consuming trips to the welfare office. The physician must plan his services according to a more or less voluminous "Book of Rules" describing the types of services and the fees allowed. To obtain payment he must apply for an "order" for each case of illness to be treated, for the care to be provided, and for the type, amount, and period of the services he wants to give. He has to fill out form after form for authorization and send in itemized bills which often have to be notarized. Forms are the bugbear of the doctor and nothing annoys him more than time-wasting paper work. The compensation he finally receives often seems to him disproportionate to the demands on his professional skill and the effort spent on form filling, bookkeeping, and accounting. The public agency which wants to compensate the physician according to the amount of service actually rendered must employ professional and clerical personnel for the approving of service; the reviewing, auditing, and certifying of each bill submitted; the regular payment of accounts; and the professional supervision of the quality of the physician's work. This means that complicated, cumbersome, and costly administrative machinery has to be maintained. Even if a special fee schedule is agreed upon, the free-choice system is more expensive and harder to budget than others. If the fees are set much below the ordinary the physicians are likely to grumble. If the total amount of allocations for a certain period of time is fixed, prorating of payments may often become necessary. This is certain to antagonize the doctors and might induce them to bill the patients for the difference to be paid "later."

Under the part-time or full-time district physician system the needy sick usually are provided with care in the home and occasionally with service at the clinic or office of the physician. The physician can render the services deemed necessary without applying for authorization and submitting itemized bills. He can count on an income that is certain and not reduced by expenses for overhead. The public agency can establish definite qualifications for the employment of physicians, set standards of service, organize the cooperation of general practitioners and specialists, administer the plan easily and inexpensively, and rely on the counsel of professional men familiar with the socio-economic conditions in the various districts. It may find the system comparatively economical. More service may be bought for the money spent and considerable savings of administrative expenses can be achieved. On the other hand, the district physician system implies that the patient cannot choose his doctor. He is, of course, free to seek the services of any physician willing to attend him without compensation. The vast majority of the physicians in private practice are excluded from participation in the program, although work may be spread by adoption of a rotating schedule. Continuity and consistency of service is not easy to maintain if Doctor A is responsible for home care, Doctor B for clinic care, and Dr. C for hospital care.

In actual practice, the district physician system often has been discredited by poor organization reflecting the "traditional niggardly attitude toward any type of service for the poor" [49] rather than by inherent shortcomings.

Those interested in the job may be very young physicians looking for a springboard into private practice and quitting as soon as they are settled; old physicians ready to retire but anxious to retain a source of income; men who have been a failure in private practice; bootlickers; or "favorite sons" of politicians. The number of district physicians appointed may be insufficient to meet the normal needs, including emergency and night calls, and entirely inadequate to cope with occasional heavy demand for service. The compensation offered may be as low "as the traffic will bear" and too low to attract well-qualified general practitioners, not to speak of accredited specialists. Tenure in office may depend on the physician's capacity to keep his mouth shut. The whim of the administrator, the wishes of a political figure, or the pressure of an influential group may prevent the district physician from doing his work with integrity and objectivity. Where such conditions prevail the patient is likely to receive inferior, hasty, or superficial service carrying the taint of relief, if not of class medicine. The conscientious physician, overworked and underpaid, is exploited and looked down upon by his colleagues. "He must be a poor doctor because he is a doctor for the poor." The agency in charge is discredited. The taxpayer has to foot the bill for mistakes and negligence. Ill-organized and cheap medical care is always costly.

If full-time salaried physicians are employed to attend the needy at the home, clinic, and hospital the patient can expect complete, continuous, and consistent service. The physician receives an income that is fair, certain, and predictable. Freed from the necessity of chasing after the elusive dollar in private practice, he can spend all his time and energy on his job. The public agency can integrate and easily administer all services for persons eligible for public medical care. Moreover, it can assign full-time physicians to take charge of certain preventive health services in addition to the care of the needy sick and thereby simplify and improve its total program. It finds no great difficulty in securing the services of competent doctors since the duties to be performed, particularly the work in the hospital, and the conditions of employment are comparatively attractive. Added advantages are the substantial economies afforded by the system and the possibility of promoting high standards of service by appointing qualified physicians through competitive examination, providing for tenure and promotion on the basis of a merit system, and supervising the adequacy of the work.

The unavoidable disadvantages of this method of organization are basically the same as those of the district physician system. The arguments advanced against it rest on evidence of many unsound administrative procedures in organizing and staffing the service; on the premise that a monthly salary check would "kill all incentive" to be interested in the patient; and on the fear that large-scale "socialization of the profession" inevitably would follow successful experience with a miniature program.

In a clinic worthy of the name those needy sick who are not bedridden can obtain thorough and competent diagnosis and treatment, both medical and social. There are readily available the services of physicians, specialists as well as general practitioners, and of nurses, medical social workers, and technical personnel; equipment for diagnostic and therapeutic procedures; and an administrative machinery geared to the needs of persons with small or no means. The physician has the essential resources in material and personnel at his disposal for full and prompt use. He is stimulated and benefited through steady and close contact with other colleagues and especially the various specialists and consultants; relieved from certain routine functions and clerical work; enabled to attend a considerable number of patients in a convenient way; and provided with an opportunity to gain experience, do research work, and participate in teaching. From the community point of view the clinic system serves to offer a wide range of specialized services; foster quality of care; keep the costs of the service relatively low by full utilization of available personnel and equipment; provide for health education in combination with care of the sick; and integrate medical care and social work.

The basic objection to clinics as they are operated now is that patients have to go there rather than to physicians in private practice if and as long as they are in need, but are not accepted and advised to seek private physicians' service when they are earning a modest living. This policy causes dissatisfaction among the sick who are shifted around as their income changes; bitterness among the physicians who lose old and can hardly gain new patients; and gaps in the service for the sick as neither continuity nor completeness of care are assured. Besides, sins of commission and omission in organizing clinic service have furnished much material for opposition to the system as such. The institution may be overcrowded and understaffed with the result that the patients, confused and anxious, have to wait for hours in inadequate rooms only to get "rush medicine." The staff may consist of young doctors, interns and medical students—all working without the supervision of experienced men. It may change so often that the patient sees a different doctor on each visit. Highly qualified physicians giving a certain part of their time to work at treatment clinics may be late or irregular at the sessions since they cannot help putting private practice before a service expected to be donated. The sick individual may be shuttled from one clinic division to another or from one clinic to several others without receiving integrated treatment. He may incur considerable expenses for transportation, spend hour after hour at each clinic, and lose precious working time. Why, he wonders, is it not possible to obtain at least the most frequently needed services at one place, and why are evening sessions for those who can keep at work so rare or even missing? Unsympathetic attitudes on the part of medical or nonmedical personnel may hurt the feelings of the patient and leave with him the impression that a "charity case" after all must be thankful for the privilege of free or low-cost medical care. "A gift-horse should not be looked in the mouth." Unintelligent or negligent organization of follow-up work, and failure to coordinate clinic, home, and hospital care may seriously impair not only the potential value of the clinic but also the effectiveness of the whole treatment program for the needy.

Visiting Nurses' Service

Originally, organization of bedside nursing of the sick in the home was left mainly to voluntary effort. Only a few public agencies took active part in the development of such service, usually by subsidizing visiting nurse associations and sporadically by employing full-time nurses of their own.

With the introduction of public health nursing a definite pattern of public policy developed. A rapidly growing number of official agencies appointed public health nurses and, thereby, accepted responsibility for an organized community service designed to give assistance in all phases of community health. This trend was greatly accelerated by the allocation of Federal funds to the states for extension and improvement of public health work under the terms of the Social Security Act of 1935. Before the war nearly three fourths of all public health nurses held full-time positions with governmental agencies. Many of them, however, were engaged in specialized work.

The old policy of utilizing available nongovernmental nurse power has not been discarded. On the contrary, it has been applied in a much improved way. Many public agencies have made more or less formal agreements with a visiting nurse association, and in some instances also with private duty nurses, concerning their cooperation in the care of needy patients with acute and chronic illnesses, the amount and period of service allowed, and the specific functions to be performed. Service authorized by the public agency is paid per visit, per hour, per day, per case, or at a set annual rate, the first method being favored lately.

In some cities a duplicate system of nursing service exists. One is maintained by one or several public agencies. The other is organized by a voluntary organization which receives tax funds for service rendered to designated groups of individuals and relies on other sources of income for service to persons not accepted for public medical care.

If properly organized, bedside nursing in the home can go far to meet the needs of women after delivery, the sick with minor acute illnesses, patients with chronic illnesses who are not seriously incapacitated, and convalescents discharged from the hospital. Medical attendance, at least after the first visit of the nurse, is required to determine the medical indication for the service, give necessary treatment, and supervise the progress of the case. Equally important are environmental conditions conducive to effective nursing. The attainment of these principles has made progress in many areas but has been seriously hampered in some communities where home medical care for the needy is not yet organized.

The public health nurse has a broad responsibility going much farther than giving nursing care to the sick and injured in the home. It is now recognized that health supervision of supposedly healthy individuals is as necessary as nursing of the sick; that education and guidance of the healthy in the essentials of personal hygiene and the intelligent use of available services is as important as instruction of the patient on pertinent medical, socio-economic, and psychological questions; and that case-finding and follow-up by trained personnel are basic to the efficacy of health service.

To attain the goal of complete service there would be needed at least one public health nurse for every 2,000 persons. Early in 1942, however, the actual ratio was one public health nurse for about 6,350 persons.[50] What was even worse, the available nurse power was distributed very unevenly. Urban areas in general compared favorably with others, although some cities were without a single public health nurse. Rural areas ordinarily fell far short of standards, and many hundreds had no public health nurse at all.

Under such conditions the public health nurses employed find it next to impossible to carry out all their duties. They cannot help but make a bitter choice. Either one basic function has to be neglected, or both can be performed but superficially. Moreover, a high degree of specialization both of service and administration in many of the larger cities presents a formidable obstacle to the utilization of available personnel for bedside care.

Hence, in some communities educational work has made great strides, but bedside nursing has made little progress. In other communities, the reverse has happened. Only in the larger cities and a few counties has a fairly complete service been made available.

As public health nursing grew, an old issue became acute: Is the knowledge, skill, and time of a highly trained professional worker necessary to satisfy the various requirements of the sick or is a division of labor between professional worker and auxiliary personnel justifiable and feasible?

Students of the subject have often expressed the opinion that systematic employment of semiskilled persons for the performance of strictly defined and relatively simple functions might serve to meet the needs of a certain number of the sick and at the same time free the public health nurse for other aspects of the work for which she is indispensable. Accepting this reasoning some agencies have established programs under which a few practical nurses and partly trained attendants, such as nurses' aides or home medical aides, carry out routine work under the direction and supervision of the graduate nurses.

Going a step farther, some organizations have supplemented home nursing by visiting housekeeper service. It is designed to maintain the household of the family prior to, during, and after the delivery of the mother; during the period of temporary disability of the housewife due to acute illness or convalescence; and in certain cases of chronic illness.

Lately, public agencies have begun to pay voluntary agencies for such service. What is even more significant, the Works Progress Administration assumed responsibility for projects under which women eligible for public assistance were employed as housekeeping aides in families receiving public aid. The application of this type of service to the home care of chronic patients has aroused particular interest.[51] Ample experience in foreign countries has shown that well-organized housekeeping service benefits all: the family, the health professions, and the community.[52]

The effectiveness of home nursing programs integrating the services of graduate nurses, practical nurses, nurses' aides, and visiting housekeepers depends on the availability of organized home medical care; proper selection, intelligent assignment, and close supervision of the auxiliary personnel; and coordination of the nursing program with other health and welfare services, official and voluntary.

Medical Social Service

Public policy has been slow to recognize that medical social service is an essential part of the hospital, the clinic, and any agency administering public medical care.

Medical social service was first developed in hospitals "as a service to the patient, the physician, the hospital administration, and the community, in order to help meet the problem of the patient whose medical need may be aggravated by social factors and who therefore may require social treatment which is based on his medical condition and care." [53] Among the three hospitals introducing medical social work about 1905 was a public facility, the Bellevue Hospital in New York City. By 1935, social service departments were operating in slightly more than one third of the 1,671 member institutions listed by the American Hospital Association. Since that time their number has grown. Public hospitals, special as well as general, have played an increasingly important part in this development.

The extension of medical social work to out-patient departments and, less frequently, to unattached clinics of various types constitutes another important step towards the improvement of the services for sick.[54] The number of public clinics employing medical social workers has multiplied in recent years, although there are no figures to show the speed and extent of the movement.

Since the early thirties a small but growing number of public agencies administering facilities and services for the sick, primarily welfare departments and divisions in charge of crippled children's programs, have taken medical social workers on their staff. With this an entirely new field is being opened. Social case work has been, and continues to be, the essential activity of the specially trained social worker employed in the hospital and clinic. Participation in the organization of community health services in the widest sense of the term is the function of the medical social worker attached to administrative agencies. It includes collection of factual information on medical needs and resources in the community; consultant service in formulating and setting up programs of public medical care, including case work services; guidance in operating services for the sick; establishment of a close working relation between the various official and nonofficial agencies engaged in health and welfare activities; staff education; promotion of public understanding and stimulation of community interest in organized care of the sick; and administration of certain aspects of public medical care.

How many medical social case workers should be on the staff of the hospital and the clinic? No definite answer to this question is possible. The type of conditions treated, the number of persons in need of social diagnosis and treatment, and the state of organization of health and welfare services in the community are the major factors influencing the number of medical social workers required for case work in facilities for the care of the sick.

How many medical social workers should be employed by an official agency administering public medical care? The duties and responsibilities, the case load in the office, and the amount of field work must be taken into account in determining the size of the staff. In the present stage of development any attempt to set quantitative standards would be futile.

While long-term planning is indispensable for medical social service to gain the place it ought to have in the community health program, immediate steps are necessary to overcome the growing pains of the young movement.

Medical social work as a specialized branch of social case work has developed mainly since the twenties. Only a few thousand persons possessing the professional education advocated by the American Association of Medical Social Workers were available when the outbreak of the war greatly intensified the need and multiplied the demand for qualified medical social workers. Thus, public agencies ready to accept responsibility for this type of service are facing a problem which only time can solve but which instant action toward increased and accelerated training can alleviate.

On the other hand, there are some hospital, clinic, and agency administrators who even in a period when competent personnel is at a premium use the social service largely, if not exclusively, for investigations into the financial conditions of the sick rather than for constructive case work—a policy which has long been criticized as unwise. In some instances the physicians attending hospital and clinic patients show scant interest in questions other than purely medical;

they make it difficult for the medical social worker to be their consultant in the area of social diagnosis and treatment and to help the sick towards a solution of their socio-economic and psychological difficulties. Employment of medical social workers in facilities for the sick is of little avail if proper use of their special knowledge and skill is not made.

Definition of the relationship between medical social work and public health nursing is the third problem that must be tackled. The two groups have much in common, despite the dissimilarity of their professional education. In principle they attain the same broad aims. In practice they differ a good deal in their emphasis on certain activities and their approach to specific problems. They may complement each other. But they also overlap, primarily in giving advice on personal hygiene; working toward emotional adjustments; interpreting medical orders in general and the relation of recommended services to the total treatment plan in particular; carrying out medical follow-up; suggesting the use of community resources; and arranging for aid from official and nonofficial agencies.

According to leaders in both fields the situation can be remedied by division of responsibilities according to the functions each group is best equipped to perform. Yet, plans to effect coordination of public health nursing and medical social case work have been adopted in a few communities only. With increasing clarification of the functions of the medical social case worker and the public health nurse at the local level, with improvement in the professional education of the two groups, and with the increase in the number of competent workers in both fields, the confusion over their relationship should be lessened. Whether it can be eliminated in this way is debatable.

Laboratory Service

Over the years there has developed a definite trend toward acceptance of public responsibility for provision of facilities equipped to carry out those technical procedures which are necessary to the establishment of a diagnosis. Public health laboratories, maintained by official health departments at the state level and also in large cities, have come to play an increasingly important role by the volume of work performed as well as their number. Clinical and roentgenological laboratories located in such public institutions as state and local general and special hospitals, preventive and treatment clinics, and health centers have become a strongly emphasized and steadily expanded standard service.

On the other hand, nonprofit voluntary hospitals and associations supporting clinics have provided for a large number of laboratories of various types, and in many states persons engaged in business or in the private practice of medicine have established commercial laboratories.

Thus, before the war in many sections of the country the public agencies concerned had at their disposal diagnostic laboratory services of various types that could be utilized in organizing programs of medical care for the needy. However, arrangements to this effect, except for the use of public health laboratories, had been made only in a relatively small number of states. They were incomplete or almost entirely lacking in many communities.[55]

Where public policy has moved forward it has developed a fairly distinct pattern. The diagnostic services provided by public institutions are used preferentially whenever possible. Nongovernmental laboratories also are admitted to service under programs of public medical care, provided they meet the standards set either by the state or the responsible agency.

The facilities supported out of tax funds usually are not reimbursed by public agencies administering medical care, as this would merely mean transferring taxpayers' money from one budget item to another. Voluntary hospitals and clinics, if paid for care of persons in need, receive a fixed sum, which includes the compensation for routine laboratory services, and fees for unusual, more expensive, and repeated tests. Often specific authorization of certain services is mandatory. Other clinical and roentgenological laboratories are paid agreed fees for authorized service rendered to persons in need. The routine, simple diagnostic or progress laboratory examinations completed by the physician in connection with the general care of a patient ordinarily are not paid for as such but are part of the professional service.

Well-equipped and well-staffed clinical and roentgenological laboratories are concentrated in large cities, rare in small communities, and lacking in many rural districts. Thus, public agencies in centers of population have no difficulty in arranging for adequate diagnostic service as part of their program for persons in need. In contrast, public agencies in small towns and thinly settled areas are faced with a serious problem. Not infrequently, there are laboratories in operation —but they are of inferior quality. Use of a good facility in the next city would entail considerable expenses for transportation and service, not to mention the jurisdictional difficulties involved.

Drugs and Related Supplies

In organizing the provision of drugs, dressings, and sickroom supplies for nonhospitalized persons in need, public policy has advanced along two major lines. Public facilities with a full-time or part-time staff have been developed early and relatively frequently. The services of pharmacists in private practice have been utilized in a systematic way lately and occasionally. In addition, a variety of other arrangements have been made in some communities.

At present there is a conspicuous disparity in the extent to which drugs are provided for the needy in various sections of the country. Moreover, in the same community the policies differ much, not only according to the group of beneficiaries, but also according to the type of drug required.

Under the system of public facilities drugs and related supplies are made available to persons in need through three channels: (1) a pharmacy located in a public hospital or out-patient department; (2) a pharmacy located in an unattached public clinic or other official building; (3) the state or local health department in the case of such prophylactic and therapeutic preparations as are required for the control of communicable diseases.

Where it is established policy to make use of professional personnel in private practice, public agencies in charge of medical care either contract with certain registered pharmacists licensed to practice in the respective state or open the opportunity to participate in the program to all those eligible. In such case detailed agreements are concluded, setting forth the professional requirements for participation of pharmacists; the drugs which may and may not be supplied; the procedures to be observed in carrying out the agreement; and the price schedules for prescriptions requiring compounding, prescriptions for ready-made preparations, and sundries.

In some communities, where public agencies pay out-patient departments in nongovernmental hospitals for service rendered to persons accepted for public medical care, compensation for drugs and dressings is included in a flat rate of payment. In small towns and rural areas it is not uncommon to have the physician furnish such drugs and dressings as are needed in the course of treatment. Payment for these items is made either on the basis of special price schedules or, not infrequently, considered part of the agreed fees for office and home calls.

With some exceptions, the patient obtains prescribed drugs at a designated facility if a public system is maintained, nongovernmental clinics are utilized, or contracts are made with one or a few pharmacists in private practice. He has "freedom of choice of vendor" according to an official list if all or most of the local pharmacists participate in the program.

Proper organization of drug supply for persons in need presents considerable problems.

First of all, quality and reliability of service must be assured. This requires selection of competent pharmaceutical personnel and professional supervision of their performance. Furthermore, efficacy and economy of prescription must be attained to keep the expenditures for drugs within reasonable limits without impairing the service. To set such goal is one thing, to reach it quite another. The recipients of public assistance include a fairly large number of people with chronic ailments who need more medication than the average individual. In addition, a certain number of sick persons are accepted for medical care only. Thus, public agencies responsible for medical care have to anticipate a justified demand for drugs on the part of their clients that is heavier than among other socio-economic groups. On the other hand, they have to reckon with the widespread desire for drugs. Persons receiving public assistance are not less "medicine-conscious" than their self-supporting fellow-citizens and by no means immune to blatant advertisements. Quite a few may wish to take advantage of an easily accessible service and request "just some pills." They may profoundly disagree with the physician on the justifiability of their demand. As ample experience has shown, it often requires the wisdom of a Solomon to make a just decision in such cases.

To promote effective and economical provision of drugs, public agencies have employed a large variety of organizational methods. Particular emphasis has been placed on the introduction and enforcement of procedures designed to eliminate indiscriminate use of the service and to reduce the costs of the individual prescription. Depending upon the basic policy, all or a varying combination of the following procedures are applied: (1) requirement of a prescription by an authorized physician for the initial order and each refill; (2) limitation of prescriptions to drugs listed in official formularies, such as *The United States Pharmacopœia, The National Formulary*, a manual issued by the administration, or a special schedule; (3) preferential use of selected standard drugs carried in stock; (4) distribution through public pharmacies of drugs bought wholesale at considerable discounts; (5) use of the approval system where "freedom of choice of vendor" is maintained, with authorization by a designated professional expert required either for all prescriptions or only for those not covered by a blanket permit, for expensive medications, large amounts of drugs and medical supplies, and "standing orders"; (6) discouragement of repeated small prescriptions and multiple prescriptions at a time; (7) limitation of the period for which drugs other than those needed in an emergency may be obtained; (8) obligation of the druggist to check each order presented as to conformity to the administrative rules; and (9) requirement on the part of the patient to pay a small charge for each service.

Appliances

In recent years there has appeared a tendency to substitute systematic arrangements for the old haphazard practices in providing appliances, including eyeglasses, for the needy. This change in policy has been brought about by the recognition of the special need for such a service among the various groups accepted for public medical care.

In general, the type of appliance has been given primary consideration in selecting the method of organizing the service. At present, simple and inexpensive medical and surgical appliances are furnished either through public pharmacies or through private druggists on the basis of special arrangements. Surgical, orthopedic, and prosthetic appliances which must be made to order ordinarily are made available through approved business firms. With them agreements are concluded concerning their cooperation in taking measurements, estimating costs, fitting, and adjustments; the specifications for various types of appliances; the price schedule; and the administrative procedures to be followed. Under this system there is either "freedom of choice of vendor" or choice from among a list of selected commercial companies and professional personnel.

The problems to be met and the principles actually applied in organizing the provision of appliances, including eyeglasses, are much like those in the related field of drug supply. However, some points deserve special mention.

Authorization of the service is the rule rather than the exception. In communities with well-organized programs of public medical care, appliances costing more than a certain amount or all those made to order are allowed only if certain requirements are met. The attending physician must make a written recommendation stating in detail the diagnosis, treatment plan, type of device suggested, and precise purpose for which it is required. The aim may be to correct a defect or deformity, secure employment, or enable the patient to attend his usual tasks. A specialist must review the case on the basis of the data submitted or an examination of his own if necessary, and recommend, in writing, approval of the request. The social service records as well as the medical records of the public agency must show that the expenditure is justifiable from all points of view. In addition, re-examination of an authorized appliance as to proper fitting and satisfaction is prerequisite to payment.

To improve the provision of eyeglasses some public agencies have formulated principles for the cooperation of the general practitioner with the ophthalmologist and of the physician with the optometrist and optician. Examinations for refractions are performed either by a medical specialist or a duly licensed and specially approved optometrist ("panel optometrist"), depending upon the recommendation made by the attending physician. After the need for eyeglasses is established and a written prescription of an authorized expert is approved by the public agency, the patient may take the order either to an optician on the official list, a designated store, or a public facility.

On the whole, current practices in providing necessary appliances leave much room for improvement. Supervision as to adequacy and economy of service is sadly lacking, despite the growing demand and the mounting expenditures for appliances.

CARE IN CLINICS, HOSPITALS, AND CUSTODIAL INSTITUTIONS: ORGANIZATION AND PAYMENT

The question of satisfactory organization of care for the needy in clinics, hospitals, and custodial institutions is closely bound up with fundamental principles of social philosophy, economics, and organization of medical practice. Of the many issues involved two are of uppermost importance: Should only governmental or also nongovernmental facilities be utilized for service to the needy at public expense? What should be the part of the clinic, hospital, and custodial institution in the total program for persons receiving public medical care?

These problems, long smoldering, became burning under the impact of the economic depression of the thirties. Since that time a growing number of communities have tried to solve them. The lines of approach chosen are quite similar in principle although they differ in detail.

Full utilization of public facilities has been the primary aim of public policy. In addition, use of tax funds to pay, where indicated, nongovernmental facilities for service rendered to the needy has been widely, although not generally, accepted as a sound principle. The development of administrative procedures for the most effective and economical utilization of various facilities according to the needs of the individual, while still in an early stage in general, has been emphasized in some advanced communities.

Clinic Care

"It is taken for granted as a sound principle of public policy that full use should be made of all governmental out-patient services existing in a community; and that where existing facilities are insufficient, governmental general hospitals should be encouraged to develop out-patient departments." [56] In essence this statement expresses the idea that public facilities should be utilized first in providing care at public expense. Actually, such a policy has long been followed in many communities, primarily in large cities.

As has been shown in Chapter Three, public clinics have not been established in numbers sufficient to meet even the most urgent needs, nor have all those in operation been equipped to offer all the essential specialized services. By necessity, the voluntary out-patient departments and unattached treatment clinics had to, and did, provide much of the care for the needy. Yet, although they relieved official agencies from expenses for the establishment and operation of facilities of their own, for a long time they received no payment or only allocations quite disproportionate to the amount of their work for "public charges." If there were any relations between public agencies responsible for medical care and voluntary clinics, they were strained by constant disputes over the extent and the manner in which payment for service to the needy should be made. Public policy, thus, was as simple as it was unrealistic. The burden of supporting services for those who could not afford private care was shifted from the taxpayer to the nongovernmental facility, only to be shifted back to those taxpayers who were ready to cover the clinics' chronic deficit by their donations.

An entirely new direction of public policy became apparent with the introduction of plans for the systematic use of tax funds to pay nongovernmental clinics for the care of the needy. Pertinent recommendations, based on the experience in a number of localities, were officially adopted in 1939 by the American Hospital Association and the American Public Welfare Association.[57] However, the spirit of cooperation, so strongly emphasized and so successfully displayed by the two national organizations, was slow to permeate the crust of indifference that had accumulated at the local level over the years. Where it did, formal agreements were concluded between the public agency and local voluntary clinics meeting definite standards. "Approved" clinics were assured of payment for such service as was authorized by the official agency. Before the war, the welfare departments in a few communities paid for more than one fourth of all visits to the participating clinics.

Significant as this course of public policy is from a general point of view, it has not yet led to the much needed coordination of all efforts, governmental and nongovernmental. Utilization of all adequate clinics in the community according to the functions they are best equipped to perform is the exception rather than the rule.

In recent years many public agencies have taken steps to develop a more equitable plan for paying nongovernmental clinics for service to the needy.[58] The old policy of allotting a lump sum has been more and more abandoned in favor of the "per-visit method of payment," which relates the compensation to the volume of service actually rendered.

Since the "visit" is the unit of reimbursable service, this term must be interpreted uniformly so as to avoid friction between the contracting parties. The American Hospital Association [59] and the United States Children's Bureau [60] have worked out pertinent definitions and also recommendations as to the procedure in counting and reporting.

In general, a clinic visit is defined as the occasion of treatment or any personal professional service for a patient.

Compared with the selection of a more adequate method of payment, the determination of a reasonable rate of pay proved to be about as difficult as tightrope walking. The clinic expected the compensation to cover at least the actual costs of service to the needy. The public agency, recognizing the justification of this demand, requested a system of cost accounting which would clearly separate expenses for the care of the needy from others, particularly those for research and teaching. Since uniform methods of computing costs are hard to introduce and, in addition, the organization and standards of various clinics in the same community differ considerably, it should not come as a surprise that the outcome of numerous and lengthy rate negotiations usually disappointed both the voluntary clinics and the public agencies. However, in a small number of communities some progress has been made. Uniform rates, while admittedly not ideal, have been adopted, and they have been set not too far below the average actual costs per visit. A tendency has appeared to simplify the administrative work by substituting inclusive rates for basic rates plus payment of "extra" services.

Inclusive rates cover either all or a varying combination of such auxiliary services as clinical laboratory tests, X-ray examinations, dressings, and ordinary drugs. As a general rule, specific authorization of the clinic service by the public agency is a prerequisite for obtaining payment. Not infrequently, review and reauthorization are required after a certain period of time or a stated number of visits, and special authorization is necessary for selected services involving considerable costs.

The most vexing problem confronting public policy today is not whether clinics for the care of the needy should be maintained, but which function they should perform in the total program of public medical care as it stands.

For a long time the opinion has been advanced that all services for the ambulatory sick in need should be concentrated in clinics which also should be responsible for care of the patient in his home. This method of organization has been chosen, for instance, in Ireland. There it was introduced as early as the first half of the nineteenth century and greatly expanded under the terms of the Medical Relief Charities Act of 1851.

In the United States, many of the larger communities, in assuming responsibility for the care of the needy, from the very beginning urged or required the use of clinics whenever feasible, without, however, developing home care as routine function of the clinics. This school of thought has continued to draw followers in many sections of the country. A typical example is the following statement in the Massachusetts *Manual of Public Assistance:*

Boards of Public Welfare should require dependent persons to take advantage of service rendered by clinics, dispensaries and out-patient departments whenever possible and desirable, and should endeavor to have agreements with clinics regarding dependents whom they refer for diagnosis and treatment.[61]

In striking contrast to those who believe clinics should be the principal facilities for the needy to obtain medical care, a second group asserts that a redefinition and restriction of the clinic functions is imperative. This school of thought maintains that the development of organized home and office care on the basis of agreements with physicians in private practice makes it possible to provide the needy with much of the service hitherto given by the clinic only. While abolition of the clinic as such is not proposed by the large majority—although it is advocated by extremists—limitation of its "sphere of influence" is demanded. The clinic should be used mainly as a diagnostic center and "clearing house," and, in addition, as a treatment auxiliary, supplementing rather than supplanting the services given by the general practitioner and specialist in private practice. Such organization is in process of development in some communities.

As stated in Chapter 3, the clinic problem is much too complex to be settled by a more or less artificial demarcation of the clinic's function in the total program of public medical care. Its ultimate solution depends on a new policy in regard to organization of medical practice.

General Hospital Care

Until the beginning of the third decade of this century public agencies expended tax funds for the hospitalization of persons in need primarily in governmental facilities. Occasionally, the management of city and county hospitals was handed over to entrepreneurs or to voluntary associations, such as nursing orders, for a fixed price a year. Such business relations usually were not amicable, not to mention other shortcomings. In San Francisco, for instance, it happened in 1857 that the city government denied the Sisters of Mercy their just claim for payment of their contractual services at the public hospital, whereupon many of the sick poor were removed to the streets. "Happily, the weather was fine, though a little cold during the night," as the local newspaper noted, so that the incident ended with no serious consequences to the patients.[62]

Public general hospitals even in large cities generally furnished only a fraction of the beds required for the adequate care of persons unable to pay and were rare or lacking in the great majority of small communities—a situation that still holds. (For details see Chapter 2.) Under such conditions the voluntary general hospitals in densely populated districts had to carry the greater part of the burden and those outside of urban areas practically all of the burden of serving the sick in need. For this work some received tax subsidies from local agencies and, occasionally, the state in the form of annual lump sum allocations. Some were invited to tender bids for the care of all "public charges" in the community during the fiscal year, the lowest bidder usually getting the contract. The majority, however, were not paid at all.

On the whole, tax funds, if appropriated, covered a negligible fraction of the expenses actually incurred by the voluntary hospitals in caring for persons with inadequate resources. To be paid by official agencies merely meant a moral victory for the hospital. The effect of such public policy was far-reaching.

To serve the needy in the community the voluntary general hospitals had to rely on the generosity of "merchant princes" and regular donations from the residents in general. In early times it was not uncommon to invite subscriptions from individuals and organizations in return for which they obtained the privilege of naming one or several poor persons to receive free hospitalization for a certain period of time.

Nongovernmental general hospitals without endowments from philanthropists and regular contributions from the citizenry found it impossible to accept any but an occasional patient for free or low-cost care. Most of those with income from endowments and gifts incurred substantial deficits if they tried to live up to the noble tradition of a "charitable institution." In spite of hearty response from benefactors the voluntary hospitals received much less in donations than they needed—and their needs were increasing from year to year.

The financial plight of the voluntary general hospital was so common that only its absence would have come as a surprise. That this situation gave cause for worry as early as the last century can be seen from the following remarks in the Annual Report for 1895 of the Trustees of the Massachusetts General Hospital in Boston:

> Although a private corporation, the work done by the Massachusetts General Hospital is practically that of a public institution, and without the hearty support of the public at large, it cannot continue indefinitely the public ministrations of the past.[63]

But it has been only in the last decades that the basic problem of the voluntary hospital became quite obvious. Each period of business prosperity brought with it overcrowding of nongovernmental facilities and under-occupancy of governmental ones. Each economic depression filled the tax-supported facilities operated for the needy; it emptied the semiprivate and private accommodations and overburdened the wards of voluntary hospitals, drastically reducing their income. In 1935 the general and allied hospitals maintained by nonprofit voluntary organizations reported a loss of nearly $35 for each $1,000 of expense.[64]

The long overdue reform of public policy was finally forced by the economic crisis of the thirties. It has been widely recognized since then that the use of tax funds to pay voluntary hospitals for the care of the needy is a reasonable policy, and that cooperation between public agencies and voluntary hospitals is imperative. To develop better mutual understanding between the two parties and guide public officials as well as hospital administrators, the American Hospital Association and the American Public Welfare Association officially adopted a statement of general policy concerning the use of tax funds for the care of the needy in nongovernmental hospitals and, also, offered detailed suggestions as to procedure. Apart from recommendations on the organization of payment and administrative points, the national associations emphasized three important principles that have been increasingly applied in recent years. They stressed the advantages of collective bargaining between public agencies and all local hospitals, organized in hospital councils where feasible. They proposed principles for the determination of standards for the admission of nongovernmental hospitals. "In communities in which an adequate number of beds can be furnished by hospitals on the approved list, hospitals not approved by the American College of Surgeons should not be utilized. Voluntary nonprofit hospitals should be used as far as available. Proprietary hospitals may be considered for use when local conditions require." Finally, the associations pointed to the fact that the governmental agencies which pay tax funds to the voluntary hospitals "must make necessary inspections and will require reports of services and cost." [65]

A good example of the new course of public policy is afforded by the legislation in the state of New York. The Social Welfare Law of this state requires hospitalization "in a hospital maintained by the municipality or in any other hospital visited, inspected and supervised by the board [of social welfare]." [66]

Heeding the advice of experts, most public agencies recently have decided to make the payments to voluntary hospitals for the care of the needy on the basis of service actually rendered rather than by lump sum appropriations. The "per diem method of payment" is most generally utilized, with the day of admission being counted a full day and the day of discharge or death being excluded in computing the length of stay of the patient.

In a growing number of communities inclusive rates have been substituted for multiple rates so as to eliminate waste of time, effort, and money in administering the program. Inclusive rates usually cover most or all of the charges for ward accommodation, meals and dietary service, use of operating and delivery room, general and special nursing, necessary clinical laboratory and X-ray services, routine medications and dressings, and special treatment services such as physical therapy. They exclude very expensive and rarely needed services and all but minor appliances.

To facilitate the determination of a "fair per diem rate" voluntary hospitals participating in a program of public medical care have been urged to adopt comparable or uniform methods of accounting and cost computing. However, the segregation of expenses for ward service of the needy from those for research and teaching and for in-patient service from those for out-patient care has presented difficulties that have not been completely overcome. Individual rates based on calculation of the patient-day costs of each hospital have been agreed upon in a small number of instances. Uniform rates for all local facilities have been favored on the theory that payment of a different rate for each hospital would result not only in local competition on a price basis but in a great amount of administrative work. Graded rates for groups of comparable hospitals have not been tried out.

It is a laborious task to arrive at a payment plan that would be just and acceptable to all voluntary facilities as well as the public agency administering the taxpayers' money. In a goodly number of communities the variations in the quality and organization of hospitals are so great that it is next to impossible to determine an average rate neither too low to penalize the best facilities nor too high to benefit unduly those of lower quality. Notwithstanding these obstacles progress has been made. In a small number of communities the agreed rates cover the greater part of the hospitals' expenses for the needy. In the majority of cases they are considerably below actual costs and often closer to one third than to one half of what the hospital spends on this type of service. The general trend is well exemplified by the development in North Carolina and South Carolina. In these states payments from cities and counties to voluntary hospitals assisted by the Duke Endowment rose from 36.1 per cent of the cost of each free day of care in 1930 to 51 per cent in 1941.[67]

The next problem, then, was to decide on the general principles governing the procedure in the hospitalization of the individual sick. Written request, including a medical certificate on the necessity of hospital care, and authorization of the service by the official agency are usual requirements.

The "Standard Hospital Agreement" worked out between the hospitals, the local departments of public welfare, and the State Department of Social Welfare in Rhode Island affords an interesting example of the tendency towards rapprochement between official agencies and nongovernmental facilities. The agreement covers the services to be provided by the participating hospitals; the groups eligible for care at public expense (residence restrictions are abolished); the authorization procedure; the payment arrangements (a flat rate is established); and accounting and administrative procedures.[68]

Payments from tax funds, formerly often mere tokens of appreciation, have come to contribute noticeably to the support of nongovernmental hospitals. In 1935, when definite payment plans were only beginning to operate in many parts of the country, the nonprofit voluntary hospitals of the general type (exclusive of mental, tuberculosis, and institutional facilities) received more than 10 per cent and the proprietary group more than 4 per cent of their income from tax funds. It is noteworthy that at that time certain special hospitals derived substantial benefit from cooperation with public agencies. Tuberculosis hospitals, proprietary as well as nonprofit, reported about one fourth of their income and nonprofit mental hospitals nearly one sixth of theirs as coming from tax funds.[69] By the end of 1941 the receipts of nongovernmental facilities from public agencies had increased further as both frequency and amount of payment grew.

The effectiveness of the modern general hospital depends on the proper utilization of its highly organized and costly diagnostic and therapeutic service. Proper utilization depends on the availability not only of programs facilitating early hospitalization, whenever medically indicated, but also of supplementary facilities and "extramural" services for those who according to medical judgment do not require general hospital care or do not need it any longer.

Present policies and administrative practices governing public medical care are not such as to enable the general hospital to play its full part in the constructive community health services.

In many areas the major, if not the sole, emphasis is being placed on provision of care in hospitals and out-patient departments, while little or no attention is being paid to other services. Under such conditions the hospital physicians and administrators have to choose between two evils. Either the patients are admitted according to strictly medical indication and discharged at the earliest possible moment consistent with adequacy of hospital care—regardless of the fact that there are no provisions for service outside the hospital; or the policies as to admission and length of stay are liberal, and then a substantial proportion of the beds are occupied by patients who do not require the full services of a general hospital.

In a relatively small number of communities, home, office, clinic, and hospital care are made available without discrimination. Some of the obstacles to the development of satisfactory and economical care of the sick and proper utilization of the general hospitals are thereby eliminated.

In all but a few communities there is an appalling lack of adequate special facilities for patients in the recovery period and for those chronically sick whose conditions require institutional care. Thus, the special needs of two large groups of patients are unmet. The general hospital designed, equipped, staffed, and operated primarily to serve patients with acute illnesses is also a refuge for a good many sick persons who are admitted or stay unnecessarily long chiefly because adequate housing, resources, or close relatives are lacking, and public assistance as well as public medical care are deficient. The taxpayer has to foot a bill which could be substantially reduced by use of facilities less complex and less expensive to build and operate than general hospitals.

Public general hospitals are the main victims of the failure of public policy to provide for all necessary special facilities. Many are the "catchalls" for all sorts of conditions, since most of the voluntary general hospitals accept primarily patients with acute illnesses and often only those with a certain type of disease. In some communities such a division of functions constitutes part of a formal agreement between public agencies and nongovernmental hospitals for the care of the needy sick. The voluntary facilities serve only patients with acute illnesses and conditions promising rehabilitation within a reasonable period of time. The public general hospitals, on the other hand, are utilized for the care of those with uncertain or no prospects of rehabilitation. Whether such policy is wise is open to serious doubt. Apart from creating difficulties of interpretation and administration, it turns the wheels of history back. The public general hospital built and operated according to modern standards would be relegated to a secondary place in the community health program. Ultimately it would be but a chronic disease hospital although it is entirely unsuited and too costly for this purpose.

Chronic Disease Hospitals

Chronic disease hospitals are conspicuous by their rarity. Their development has been retarded by almost universal neglect of the widespread need for adequate, humane, and economical care of the sick with long drawn-out maladies.

Patients with mental deviations, tuberculosis, and serious crippling conditions have been provided with suitable, although not always the best possible, care in specialized facilities. In contrast, other chronically sick persons in need of institutional care have been treated with little regard to their individual requirements. If they were poor and not too much incapacitated by disease, accident, or congenital defect, they were accommodated in the almshouse, that monument to degradation, or in a substandard private nursing home, that monument to neglect. Patients in need of intensive medical care for prolonged treatment, and those who grew worse or became acutely ill while in an almshouse, had to be admitted to a general hospital under government control, if there was any.

Although few public agencies were indulging in the pleasant daydream that they had done their duty to both the chronic sick in need and the community as a whole, it has been only in recent years that a new course of public policy was charted. Due to the untiring efforts of a few individuals, especially Dr. Ernst P. Boas of New York,[70] and the exhaustive study of chronic illness in New York City by Miss Mary C. Jarrett,[71] differentiated programs of institutional care for persons with chronic illness were adopted in a few communities. They are based on the recognition that age, type of disease or defect, degree of disability, and mental capacity and temperament have to be given due consideration in deciding on the types of facilities needed and in selecting patients for the institution best suited to the individual case. In 1940 a joint committee of the American Hospital Association and the American Public Welfare Association stressed that persons "in need of active and continuous treatment by a physician" and those "who need chiefly skilled care by a trained nurse" belong in a hospital and suggested various alternatives for the development of such service.[72]

The idea of converting an almshouse into a chronic disease hospital always has been appealing by its seeming simplicity. It has attracted increasing attention lately. Many almshouses became underoccupied after the introduction of special assistance programs, because the Social Security Act prohibits payments to persons residing in public institutions. But the realization of such a project proved to be beset with difficulties. While a few almshouses needed only slight improvements in physical plant, the majority required major alterations, and all of them had to be adapted to their new function by drastic changes in equipment, personnel, and management. Such steps have been taken in some states where a few large institutions have been transformed into facilities for the care of the chronically ill, and many of the smaller institutions have been closed.

The second line of approach used by some public agencies was quite different. Functional buildings were erected in which all the chronic sick of an area were concentrated. While this principle was supported by experts, details of organization were much disputed.

One school of thought favored the "integrated acute-chronic hospital plan" under which sections of the general hospital or special units on its grounds would be set aside for the chronic sick. This method of organization, it is argued, would facilitate the initial and final assignment of the new patient, his easy transfer when needed, full utilization of already available resources in equipment and specialized personnel, economical administration of all services, and easy contact between the sick and his family and friends. An integrated social, medical, educational, and research plan would have moral and scientific value and serve to avoid "the 'dumping' process by which undesirable patients are transferred from general hospitals to public institutions of less satisfactory qualifications." [73]

Admitting the feasibility of such a plan in certain cities, a second school of thought nevertheless believes that separate chronic disease hospitals offer considerable advantages. They could be built and operated less like acute hospitals and, thereby, give the chronic patient the special consideration, comfort, psychological atmosphere, occupational services, and recreational facilities he has to forego on a special ward or in a special pavilion of a general hospital. They could be staffed with personnel giving their full interest and time to the task, and develop into research and teaching centers on medical, psychological, and socio-economic problems of chronic illness. They would prevent inadequate care in small facilities by serving a region rather than a political unit with small population and be less expensive to build as they could be erected outside densely populated areas. In this age of rapid transportation, facilities located at a distance from the centers of population would be easily accessible. Actually both methods of organization have been employed, although only sporadically.[74]

Custodial Care

To provide for those chronic sick, physically handicapped, and physically and mentally infirm aged who "require only care by practical nurses or attendants, with medical and nursing supervision (so-called 'custodial care')," [75] public institutions, such as the almshouse, poor farm, or county home, have been increasingly equipped with special facilities. At present, the provisions for the sick in such institutions range from a primitive infirmary supervised by a visiting physician and served by attendants to elaborate hospital units with resident physicians, graduate nurses, and visiting specialists, including dentists.

Hospital units have been developed more recently in the large city institutions, and, in particular, in the large county homes or state institutions that have superseded small town almshouses in some sections of the country. Most of them have been steadily improved and some meet reasonable standards. In contrast, the sick wards in small institutions are distinguished by the archaic conditions under which they are operated. They are a disgrace to any civilized community.

On the whole, the public provisions for custodial care are utterly inadequate. The location of some of the facilities in buildings resembling a glorified jail does not make them attractive even to people accustomed to such an environment. In 1940 the common man still had good reason to feel as his ancestors did. "Death appears less terrible than a residence in the almshouse," as Dr. James Jackson and John C. Warren of Boston put it in 1810.[76]

To remedy the disgusting conditions prevailing in many communities, various alternatives have been suggested. They are: (1) use of private nursing homes; (2) conversion of public institutions that have become useless; (3) erection of functional buildings under public auspices.

In many parts of the country, nursing homes, operated for profit, have been utilized by public agencies for quite some time. The idea appeared tempting. The expenditure of tax funds for the building of public facilities would be saved. Simple medical, nursing, and dietary care in an environment resembling that of a family home would be provided. In practice, however, the experience often was disappointing. A surprisingly large number of nursing homes were found to have poor standards. Some were death traps rather than havens for the chronic sick. Some were more interested in handsome profits than in good service and ruthlessly exploited both patients and taxpayers. Although time and again shocking defects in certain nursing homes became common knowledge and aroused much public indignation, the responsible agencies preferred to follow the example of the proverbial ostrich. It has been only lately that a few states set minimum standards for nursing homes and enforced them through licensing and supervision, including regular inspection. A good example of this policy are the standards prescribed by the New Jersey State Department of Institutions and Agencies.[77]

In line with the newer policy in paying nongovernmental hospitals, the approved nursing homes now usually are compensated on a per diem basis for service rendered to certain recipients of public assistance. However, the rates actually paid often are so low that nursing homes anxious to maintain reasonable standards find it impossible to furnish satisfactory service and, rightfully, refuse to take more than a few "guests" at public expense.

Substandard proprietary "homes" not only have continued to be accepted by a goodly number of public agencies but are flourishing more than ever. In the absence of adequate institutions they are much used by ailing old people who pay for their care out of the grants received under old-age assistance programs.

Conversion of a public institution of the almshouse type, emptied by the development of special public assistance programs, into a home for the chronic sick in need of custodial care has been considered frequently in recent years, but carried out in a few instances only. To prevent unsatisfactory organization, the American Hospital Association and American Public Welfare Association, through a joint committee on hospital care, have worked out the minimum essentials for such homes in regard to buildings and equipment, personnel, and policies of medical administration.[78]

Ambulance Service

Although the first city ambulance service in the world was established at the Bellevue Hospital in New York City as early as 1869, transportation to and from the hospital is not yet an integral part of public provisions for the needy sick in every part of the country. Where it is organized, one of the following methods are employed: (1) a public hospital or a unit of government, usually a city or county and, occasionally, the state, maintains a fleet of ambulances; (2) the public agency pays the nonprofit voluntary hospital a fixed price for transportation of patients accepted for public medical care or includes compensation for this service in the rate paid to the institution; (3) the public agency makes a contract with a commercial firm. In addition, some public agencies pay the railroad fare for the patient and his escort.

While the importance of organized ambulance service has been recognized, the need for systematic development of inexpensive transportation to treatment clinics has been disregarded. The result is that in many areas those beneficiaries of public assistance who live in suburban districts find it hard to make use of a clinic in the center of population, and that many low-income families in rural areas shun the inconvenience and expense of a trip to a clinic in the next city where they could obtain badly needed diagnostic tests and specialists' services at low charges.

ADMINISTRATIVE ORGANIZATION

As provision of general medical care for persons in need developed from an incidental activity to a regular function of governmental agencies, its administrative organization was gradually changed. Weak spots were mended, but no attempt was made to build a new system suited to new conditions.

Administrative powers, duties, and functions were redistributed among the various levels of government. Professional direction of professional matters was instituted and special units, increasingly headed by physicians, were created in local and state agencies responsible for general programs of public medical care. Provision was made for participation of the health professions, the hospitals, and the various health and welfare agencies in the organization and operation of plans for the sick in need. Administrative procedures for the attainment of adequacy of service were introduced.

Marked as these trends in public policy were, they did not appear in all sections of the country nor in all political subdivisions of progressive states. Thus, the present picture of the administrative organization of general programs of public medical care is kaleidoscopic. It varies not only from state to state but from community to community within the same state, and even from one local agency to another.

Distribution of Administrative Responsibility

Following the English precedent the early settlers vested administrative responsibility for the medical care of the poor in small local units, such as townships or even villages. This method of organization was in line with the ideas common to the time. Support of the poor was regarded as a purely local obligation and, hence, to be financed entirely from local sources. Typical of the early policy is a decree of 1672 of the general court of the colony of Connecticut to the effect that "every town within this colony shall maintain their own poor." [79] Significantly, one exception from the general rule had to be made soon. Nonresident paupers in urgent need of medical attendance and institutional care were accepted for temporary relief, with the town of residence charged for the costs. The New England system was copied widely and later became dominant in many states.

A policy which could be defended in an agricultural society and the period of simple medical care became untenable in the machine age and the era of scientific medicine. There had grown up countless small authorities responsible for persons dependent upon public aid. Their resources proved much too meager to provide for the rapidly growing army of persons unable to pay for the many and costly services modern medicine had to offer. The small political units could not avoid strictly limiting both the number of persons accepted for medical care at public expense and the amount of service given to them. Even so, payment of a single bill for hospitalization of a patient with serious illness often absorbed the greater part of the funds set aside for relief.

The weakness of such administrative organization has been increasingly realized. A new principle of action has emerged since the nineteenth century and has been applied more frequently since the nineteen thirties. It is based on the recognition "that the geographical area from which public funds are drawn must, often, be larger than the geographical unit of administration," as Michael M. Davis has stated.[80] In various sections of the country financial responsibility for the general care of persons in need was shifted from towns to counties, with costs to the contained civil units prorated in terms of tax assessments. Cities, however, usually were not included in such redistribution of duties and functions. Kansas was one of the states adopting such legislation in the second part of the nineteenth century.

Going a step farther some states designated the county as the principal administrative unit responsible for operation of general programs of public medical care, although they did not entirely abolish the principle of township responsibility.

The creation of unified and financially stronger administrative units at the local level constituted but one of several recent measures for the adaptation of the administrative structure to modern requirements. In 1941, Mr. Justice Byrnes summed up contemporary concepts on distribution of government responsibility by declaring: "Recent years, and particularly the past decade, have been marked by a growing recognition that in an industrial society the task of providing assistance to the needy has ceased to be local in character. The duty to share the burden, if not wholly to assume it, has been recognized not only by State governments, but by the Federal government as well." [81]

The state has long participated in the administration of general medical care for persons in need. Until a few decades ago, however, its powers, duties, and functions were kept within close boundaries. In many sections of the country the state had financial responsibility for the care of persons without settlement, the "non-inhabitants," later often called state paupers. This policy dated back to colonial times. As early as 1750 it was put on the statute books that colony aid was to be provided "to all unsettled sick paupers whether their sickness was of an infectious nature or not." [82] Furthermore, the state maintained general hospitals, special hospitals, and custodial institutions, subsidized local hospitals rendering service to the poor, or did both. Finally, it exercised some supervision over political subdivisions, originally through courts and later through special boards.

In the last two decades the situation has changed notably. The principle of local responsibility for the administration of general medical care for persons in need has been maintained, except in a few states and territories. But many states have assumed broader responsibility in this field.[83] In so doing they have followed quite different courses, though. The result is a confusing multiplicity of actual practices, some dating back to old times, some established in recent years. On the one extreme are some state agencies acting merely in a consultant capacity upon invitation. On the other extreme are several state and territorial agencies vested with complete legal, financial, and administrative responsibility for the operation of a direct service program. In between are two groups of states pursuing totally dissimilar policies. One group confines its responsibility to the support of selected services, mainly general hospital and out-patient care in state controlled and/or local facilities and, in some instances, also home and office care, including provision of personnel, equipment, and supplies. The other group, comprising a growing number of states, emphasizes the systematic development of state-local cooperation by clear definition and division of administrative powers, duties, and functions.

Where general medical care for persons other than beneficiaries of special assistance is organized on the basis of state-local cooperation, the central agency performs some or all of the following functions: formulation of the broad policies as to organization and administration of public medical care within the state; establishment of standards for the selection of facilities and personnel, both professional and administrative, and for the installation and operation of programs in the localities; general promotion of local activities; provision of consultant service to local agencies in establishing and administering their own plans; financial assistance to local programs; and general supervision of local plans.

The localities, on the other hand, have full responsibility for the organization, support, and management of their own program according to local needs and conditions. They receive financial aid from the state for designated expenses, provided their plan meets the requirements set by the state.

In sharing the costs of general medical care with political subdivisions some states have continued time-tested practices. They collect from local units for care rendered to needy persons in state-controlled facilities or pay local institutions for service to certain groups of patients. Other states have adopted schemes by which the total costs of an inclusive program are divided between state and local units according to a prearranged schedule.

The principle of reimbursement of localities for specified expenditures, already uniformly adopted for special assistance programs, has been used by a few states to promote medical care for recipients of general assistance and medically needy persons. This new direction of public policy is well exemplified by the law of Rhode Island.

The Rhode Island General Public Assistance Act of 1942 declares that "the state shall reimburse cities and towns not less than 70 per cent of any assistance granted under the provisions of this article, and also not less than 70 per cent of the ordinary and necessary administration costs incurred." [84] (The provisions include medical care.)

Adoption of the policy of state reimbursement of local expenditures must not be construed as implying uniformity in procedure. Actually, great disparity prevails in regard to both the conditions of qualification for reimbursement and the percentage to which services and charges are reimbursed. To guide local agencies through the numerous and diverse rules, the New York State Department of Social Welfare has issued the detailed *Analytical Chart of Reimbursable Medical, Dental and Nursing Care.*

Since the adoption of the Social Security Act the Federal government has participated in the development, improvement, standardization, and financial support of state programs for special assistance groups. But it has been unable to take constructive action in regard to medical care, as existing legislation is not suited to such purpose. According to the wording of the Social Security Act funds used by the states to furnish assistance to needy individuals can be matched by the Federal government only in so far as the assistance takes the form of unrestricted money payments. Federal reimbursement is not possible if expenditures are made in the form of direct payments from the agency in charge to professional persons or institutions rendering service. Thus, a unique situation has been created. States which are anxious to obtain Federal reimbursement of expenses for the care of sick recipients of special assistance have to pay the beneficiary some cash benefit, although they know perfectly well that all too often such allowances are insufficient for the purpose or spent unwisely. States which provide for service adequate to meet the needs of the sick are penalized, as they cannot claim Federal reimbursement for the expenses incurred.

The principle of Federal-state cooperation has not been extended to programs of general assistance, except for the brief period from 1933 to 1936 when the Federal Emergency Relief Administration was in operation. Thus, the states and local communities have to bear the full costs of medical care for recipients of general assistance and the medically needy.

Professional Direction of Public Medical Care Programs

In the first phase of development, lay persons such as overseers of the poor, justices of the peace, county supervisors, and judges of the county courts were exclusively responsible for administration of public medical care for the poor. In particular, they decided over eligibility for service and determined the type, amount, and period of care.

The overseers of the poor occupied a key position in the local administration of relief, including medical care, ever since the passage of the early poor laws, such as those of Pennsylvania (1771) and the Northwest Territory (1790 and 1795). In many sections of the country, they have continued to control the provision of medical care. In North Dakota, for instance, legislation of 1933 and 1935 listed among the duties of the overseers of the poor the following:

> The overseer of the poor in each county commissioner's district shall . . . in cases of necessity, promptly provide medical and surgical attention for all the poor in his district, who are not provided for in public institutions and shall see that such medicines as prescribed by the physician or surgeon in attendance upon the poor, are furnished, provided that in counties where a county physician or physicians have been appointed on an annual salary, the overseer of the poor shall call upon the nearest county physician to attend such poor person in need of certain medical or surgical attention.[85]

It has been long recognized that some personal qualifications are necessary for an administrator serving the underprivileged and entrusted with the sacred duty of spending taxpayers' money. Significantly, several early acts, such as that passed in Detroit in 1809, required "discreet persons" to be appointed. But until quite recently public policy has been adamant to the idea of utilizing professional advice, assistance, and direction in the administration of public medical care.

Prejudice against the expert, that venerable tradition of public administration, still persists. In a number of states persons wholly unfamiliar with the basic principles of modern health policy decide on the acceptance of applicants and the service to be granted; the judges of the county courts are charged by law with the determination of eligibility of "indigent persons"; and "court commitments" are required before treatment can be given to certain groups, such as crippled children.

Defects other than absence of medical participation were characteristic of the old administrative organization of public medical care for the poor. At best, the executives were public-spirited citizens accepting service with the official agency as a side line, and the staff was composed of sincere persons with good intentions and no special training. At worst, the appointees were chosen for their political affiliation. In many a community administration of public medical care came to be regarded as the happy hunting ground for the incompetent with good connections; the office of the executive degenerated into a petty political job; and the incumbents left behind them an unsavory record of mismanagement. Reviewing the development up to the middle of the thirties, Michael M. Davis listed as the outstanding weak point in administration of public medical care "political influence upon the selection of patients, the appointment of personnel, and the methods of institutional administration." [86]

Since the early thirties a trend has appeared to provide for professional participation in the administration of public medical care for persons in need. In 1939 the American Public Welfare Association stressed that "medical programs should be under the direction of qualified salaried medical officers of the governmental authority, who should be appointed on the basis of merit." [87] At that time only a few of the agencies in charge of general programs of medical care employed physicians in executive positions. But their number has grown since. Agencies in larger cities and the more densely populated counties have tended to appoint full-time medical administrators selected through competitive examination, while those in smaller communities have increasingly secured the services of part-time medical consultants. In line with this policy special administrative units, often called division of medical care, have been set up in a number of agencies. In some instances they are staffed with physicians, dentists, pharmacists, and medical social workers as well as clerical personnel.

In most of the cities and counties and also within the state governments these divisions were established in welfare departments. Such a course of action was chosen for several reasons. Welfare departments had long been administering such medical care of needy persons as was not provided under special programs for the control of certain diseases. Vested by statute with the power and duty to operate public assistance plans, they had not only the right but the duty to administer all benefits and services paid with assistance funds. The welfare departments provided for such essentials of life as shelter and food, needed by the large majority of applicants as badly as medical care. They knew already most of the sick unable to pay for their own care and, thus, could provide for them without time-consuming and effort-wasting determination of eligibility.

The recent trend of public policy is well exemplified by the development in New York. In that state the administrative rules governing public medical care for the needy require delegation of "the direction of the medical aspects of the plan to a licensed physician." [88] In Nassau County, New York, the official rules state: "Administrative responsibility for the authorization of all types of medical care is delegated by the Commissioner of Public Welfare to the Division of Medical Care," and "The Medical Director shall be a Doctor of Medicine, licensed in the State of New York, qualified by Civil Service examination and appointed by the Commissioner to serve on a salary basis, with administrative authority for the Medical Care Program of the Department of Public Welfare." [89]

Health departments have but very rarely taken over the administration of some or all services for the sick in need. It is noteworthy that in 1939 the Tennessee legislature passed an act creating a separate "Medical Care Division" in the State Department of Public Health "to improve and regulate in a better manner the expenditure of funds . . . for medical care or medical services of every sort. . . ." [90]

In general, public health circles have been unwilling to accept general medical care as a field for development, although they have been most active in the promotion of special programs including treatment. As Joseph W. Mountin remarks "their attitude in large measure is closely related to the evolution of the public health program." [91] Sanitation of the environment, control of communicable diseases, and health education have been successively brought into the scope of public health activities, while general medical care has remained outside. The health officers, however, have a weighty reason for their reluctance. They fear administration of all tax-supported care of the sick would absorb so much of their time that the preventive health services would suffer, or primary emphasis on the traditional functions would make it impossible to give more than perfunctory service to administration of medical care. In addition, some are disinclined to hold the purse string for another agency, and some are afraid of jeopardizing their relation with the medical profession.

Obviously, some of the arguments offered by public welfare and public health circles in support of the present administrative organization of public medical care rest on grounds that are untenable. Others will lose much of their weight as tax-supported services increase and other payment methods are developed. This whole question will be discussed in detail in connection with the problem of planning for administrative organization. (See Chapter Six.)

The duties of the medical administrators in welfare departments vary a good deal, depending upon the type of agency and its responsibilities and the willingness of the administration to recognize the province of the physician. In general, the physician is autonomous in matters involving medical judgment, treatment, and medical standards. In well-organized local agencies he advises the administration in planning and developing organized medical care; directs the professional aspects of the program in operation; determines medical needs by passing on applications; reviews and audits medical bills where the panel system is in use; provides for follow-up of patients, primarily those needing prolonged or high-cost treatment; coordinates the various services, medical and social; supervises the adequacy of facilities and services; and acts as liaison officer between his own department and the local health professions, facilities, and health and welfare agencies. If he serves on a part-time basis, he is not permitted to attend patients for whom the agency pays the bill, although this wise rule is not generally observed.

The need for administrative coordination of medical care and social work has been fully recognized in advanced states. In New York State, for instance, a local plan, to be approved, must meet the following requirements:

The plan must provide for: (a) the use of physicians to determine the medical needs of any person applying for medical care; (b) the use of social workers to determine financial eligibility of such person for care at public expense; (c) informing social workers of the medical and social needs of the applicant, and for joint planning between medical and social workers where there is an interdependence between the treatment and social factors in the case. . . .[92]

The major duties of the medical advisor or medical director of a state welfare department are: (1) to advise the administration on administrative policies, standards, and procedures relating to medical care; (2) to organize the facilities and the medical and allied personnel necessary for service to the sick in need; (3) to direct the operation of the medical care program of the state or promote the development of local programs, as the case may be; (4) to assemble the necessary statistical data and initiate and supervise studies pertaining to the operation of state or local programs; (5) to serve as consultant to the various agencies providing for medical care; (6) to act as liaison officer between his own agency and other state agencies engaged in health service, the organizations representing the professions and hospitals at the state and local levels, and individual members of the professions.

Advisory Committees

In contrast to earlier times when the administration of public medical care for the poor was hidden from the outside world behind a Chinese Wall, welfare departments in various sections of the country recently have begun to secure the advice and assistance of the health professions, hospitals, and various official and nongovernmental health and welfare agencies in the planning and administration of service for persons in need.

Advisory committees representing the various professional groups and organizations concerned have been formally established by governmental agencies at the state as well as the local levels, although up to the beginning of the war only in the minority of the authorities responsible for medical care programs. This trend is illustrated by the following examples:

The Chicago Relief Administration, in addition to its general health advisory committee, has appointed technical advisory committees of physicians, dentists, and druggists, each committee consisting of persons nominated by the respective professional society.

A Michigan law of 1941 authorized the county boards to appoint "an advisory committee consisting of 1 doctor of medicine, nominated by the county medical society; 1 dentist, nominated by the district dental society; and 1 druggist, nominated by the district pharmaceutical association, to assist in formulating policies of medical care and auditing and reviewing bills for same." [93]

Recognizing the importance of active cooperation of all groups and agencies concerned, several states have given a voice in state advisory committees to representatives of the various agencies engaged in health service and the public at large as well as the health professions. The following examples will serve to show pertinent details.

In the state of Washington a State-Medical-Dental Board has been created in connection with the introduction of a medical care program for recipients of old-age assistance. It has ten members: four physicians recommended by the State Medical Association; two dentists recommended by the State Dental Association; and one representative each of the State Nurses Association, State Hospital Association, State Department of Health, and State Department of Social Security.

In Indiana a state advisory committee on medical aid has been appointed by the State Department of Public Welfare. It includes three representatives of the medical profession and one representative each of the dentists, pharmacists, public health nurses, hospitals, State Board of Health, State University Medical Center, judges' association, and the lay public.[94]

The functions of these advisory committees vary, depending upon the organization of the medical division in the welfare department. Where a medical director is appointed, the committee advises and assists in (1) formulating broad policies as to organization, development, and improvement of medical care; (2) setting standards of service; (3) determining qualifications of personnel and facilities; (4) selecting methods of paying the health professions and facilities; (5) maintaining standards of service; and (6) supervising compliance of the participating individuals and facilities with the terms agreed upon. Where there is no medical director the advisory committee performs additional functions, such as suggesting appropriate procedures in dealing with individual cases, deciding on "incapacity," and reviewing bills.

As a general rule, the ultimate decision over policy and procedures as to organization and administration rests with the public agency.

Adequacy of Service

Establishment and maintenance of adequacy of service is one of the foremost responsibilities of public agencies providing medical care. To attain this goal a variety of interrelated administrative procedures must be adopted. They include:

1. Determination of standards as to type, scope, amount, period, and accessibility of service; selection of professional and auxiliary personnel for both direct service and administrative work; and selection of institutional facilities

2. Provision at public expense of consultant, specialist, and diagnostic services for the practicing members of the various health professions

3. Supervision of medical care facilities, health personnel, and medical care programs as to quantitative and qualitative adequacy of service

4. Coordination of medical care and social work

In the preceding sections of this chapter frequent references have been made to newer administrative procedures designed to raise the standards of public medical care for persons in need and coordinate organized care of the sick with social work. While the special services, in particular the crippled children's programs, have made great strides toward the goal of adequacy, the general programs have just begun to lose the dreary connotations of the past. Much of this disparity is due to the fact that the very principles which have been generally and successfully applied to the operation of special programs have been but reluctantly used in administering general programs. One of the outstanding weaknesses of the old system of public medical care for the poor has been the lack of supervision by experts. One of the distinctive features of newer policy is the introduction of professional supervision of professional matters.

Supervision of tax-supported medical care is necessary for various reasons. High standards of service must be maintained. Completeness and continuity of care must be ensured. Maximum results must be obtained at the lowest cost consistent with adequacy. The honest, conscientious, and careful members of the health professions must be protected against those few colleagues who, unintentionally or deliberately, cause serious damage to the common plan by disregarding the established standards of service or by violating the rules of professional conduct.

There has been supervision of medical care ever since communities raised taxes to provide for the sick poor. But it was directed solely toward prevention of abuse as interpreted by the lay administrator, and it was exercised by restricting both the number of people "on the town" and the use of the meager service there was. He who spent little money was certain to be praised as an efficient administrator heeding the public mandate for economy.

That the commandment "Thou shalt not waste" can be obeyed

more humanely as well as more effectively by concentrating supervisory activities on the adequacy of the service furnished in the individual case, is a conviction that has gained ground but slowly. It may be doubted whether any human being is able to make a satisfactory adjustment between objective need and subjective desire for good medical care, between demand and available resources, and between poor man's treatment and luxury service. As a worried welfare physician once put it: "The indigent, God bless them, are not by any means the easiest people with whom to deal; they are often more demanding and unreasonable than those who can pay their way." But experts agree that an intelligently designed and reasonably executed scheme of professional supervision of public medical care can yield valuable results. Such a system provides for local supervision of both applications for medical care at public expense and services rendered by the health professions and medical care facilities. It gives the state full power to exercise general supervision over local programs. Some or all of these principles have been recently put into practice in a number of states.

In a growing number of localities applications of patients or requests of the attending physicians for treatment at public expense are first referred to the medical social worker for the necessary investigations (checking of master file or special investigation, and checking of control file) and determination of eligibility. If the case can be accepted according to the local standards, a designated physician decides on type, amount, and period of medical care.

Where service is organized on the basis of the free-choice fee-for-service system, review of all applications by the medical officer of the agency or a professional committee is common. Suffolk County in New York State, for instance, has established the following rule:

All cases requiring medical care at public expense shall be subject to review by the Department of Public Welfare or the Professional Advisory Committee or both. All records and X-rays for such cases shall be made available to the Department of Public Welfare or the Professional Advisory Committee upon request. Consultants may be employed by the Commissioner to review problem cases. . . .[95]

Following the medical decision the division of social service is informed of the care authorized, and the division of audit and control is notified of the costs.

Recognizing that professional supervision of professional services is one of the essentials of good administration, a number of agencies have taken steps to enable each profession to supervise its own field. Physicians, dentists, pharmacists, medical social workers, and, occasionally, nurses on the staff of the welfare department or special reviewing committees are charged with carrying out supervisory work.

The scope of supervision and the principal methods employed vary greatly. Not only do different systems of organizing and paying for professional services present different problems, but there is also a good deal of disagreement about the objectives to be attained. The following review is confined to administrative practices for the supervision of physicians' services. Essentially the same procedures are used to supervise the services rendered by other health professions.

Where part-time or full-time physicians are appointed for home care or various other types of care, professional supervision is focused on attainment of adequate service. Such a policy, however, can be found only in a small fraction of the cities and counties employing salaried physicians.

Where the free-choice system in combination with the fee-for-service method of payment is adopted, the supervisory procedures include one set designed to control the expenditures and another set designed to ensure quality of care. In the first group belong the following practices, some or all of which are followed in a good many communities: (1) limitation of the type, amount, and period of service through authorization of each request for treatment; (2) review of medical accounts at regular intervals, with approval of claims for allowed services and deductions for the others; (3) limitation of the monthly or annual income the individual physician may obtain from the public agency, with payments for authorized major surgery and obstetrical care excluded from consideration; (4) establishment of a common pool for payment of physicians' services, with prorating of individual accounts if the sum available for a definite period is insufficient; (5) requirement for both physician and patient to sign the treatment order and confirm the service before the bill is submitted to the agency; (6) restriction on free choice by requiring the patient to give valid reasons for a change of doctor during the same illness or within a stated period.

The method of group control through the pattern of practice set by the entire number of participating physicians has been employed in a few instances only, although its relative merits have been proved again by recent Canadian experience.[96] This technique allows to evaluate in an objective and comparatively uncomplicated way the frequency of medical attention, amount of service, type of service given, and fees claimed by the individual physician as compared with the group average.

To promote good quality of care some agencies, in cooperation with the professional groups concerned, have set the following requirements: (1) the participating members of the health professions must keep accurate records and, on request, make them available to the professional persons in charge of supervision; (2) requests for service are reviewed as to the adequacy of the proposed treatment plan; (3) selected specialists' services are subject to the decision of a consultant or the reviewing committee; (4) inspection of the quality of work performed is mandatory for designated types of service, such as dental care, and for appliances; (5) the individual physician must not accept more than a certain number of patients.

Not a few of the medical divisions and professional advisory committees, greeted with high hopes for their contribution to the improvement of medical care, have developed into something resembling a combination of a mail-order house for authorizations and an accounting office. The professional men in charge of supervision have to spend most of their time on routine work, mainly the checking of treatment requests as to compliance with the complicated provisions of the plan, and the reviewing of bills as to accuracy, completeness, and reimbursability. Small wonder that both the physicians in private practice and the medical administrators are becoming deeply disappointed. By painful experience they uncover now what has been found before: "To eliminate all barriers between the general practitioners and the relief recipients and to pay the physicians according to services rendered is a direct invitation to trouble. To hope for a satisfactory system without any form of control is to display a naive faith." [97] Cumbersome, annoying, and costly devices for the control of expenditures are the price that must be paid for the fee-for-service method of compensation and unlimited free choice of physicians.

Where supervision of general hospital care is accepted as a legitimate function of the public agency footing the bill, checking of indication for and period of hospitalization are the administrators' major activities. Medical consultants are increasingly employed for this purpose.

In general, hospitalization of patients for elective medical and surgical diagnosis or treatment at public expense is subject to prior approval of the attending physician's recommendation. If immediate hospitalization is necessary because of a genuine emergency, the hospital is required to notify the public agency within a certain period of time and to submit a report of the facts of the case, including a statement of the physician in attendance as to the necessity of immediate admission.

To control the length of stay in the hospital either of two procedures are in use. The initial authorization is limited to a definite number of days or weeks of care, and review of the case and reauthorization are required for additional treatment; or norms are set for the period of hospitalization of certain types of illness and approval of extended care must be secured if the norm is likely to be exceeded. In view of the difficulties of making a just decision from the writing desk, in particular in doubtful cases, the public agencies, participating hospitals, and medical societies in some communities have amicably settled a much debated question. According to the agreement the medical consultant may visit the patient with the consent of his doctor, review the case record, and confer with the attending physician on the problems involved; and the medical social worker may enter the hospital to procure pertinent information on socio-economic factors.

Extension of state powers to include supervision of local facilities and services for sick persons in need is one of the tendencies appearing in recent public policy.

A small but growing number of states have taken steps to establish and maintain supervisory control over the adequacy of local programs of public medical care. They formulate the general principles to be followed by the political subdivisions in drafting their own programs; require local plans to be submitted for approval before they are put in operation and declared eligible for financial aid; reimburse only services meeting the qualifications set by the central agency; and employ specialists for consultant service and supervision.

The majority of the state agencies, however, exercise only a negligible amount of supervision over local facilities and services, although most of them make regular, and in some instances considerable, allotments for the care of the needy. Noteworthy in this connection is the fact that the Social Security Board requires a supervising ophthalmologist in each state program of aid to the blind.

To determine the adequacy and efficacy of public medical care as well as its costs, annual reports on all tax-supported services are indispensable. The basic statistical data needed include the following:

1. Average number of persons receiving public assistance during the year, by type of assistance

2. Annual number of persons receiving medical care at public expense, by recipients of general assistance, recipients of special assistance, persons receiving public aid from other sources such as work relief, and persons accepted for medical care only

3. Annual number of persons whose applications for public medical care have been denied, by type of care requested

4. Annual number of persons, by categories, receiving specified care such as physicians' care (by general practitioners and specialists) at the home, office, clinic, and hospital; dental care; bedside nursing in the home; drugs; appliances; hospitalization in general and special hospitals; and custodial care

5. Annual number of specified services rendered to persons in the various categories, including number of home, office, and hospital calls of physicians; number of dentists' services (by major types); number of clinic visits (by type); number of days of care in hospitals and custodial institutions; number of drug prescriptions; and number of specified appliances furnished

6. Annual expenditures for all services and for administrative purposes, by categories of beneficiaries

7. Annual expenditures for specified services, by categories of beneficiaries

These figures constitute the minimum. Additional information would greatly contribute to the proper evaluation of the program. Data on sex and age distribution of the beneficiaries will serve to show the bearing of these factors on demand and need for medical care. Information on the illnesses treated, classified by the main diagnostic groups or types of important diseases, would furnish the key to many problems confronting administrators of health services—provided accurate and complete diagnoses can be procured.

By systematic collection, proper classification, and suitable computation * of even a limited number of statistical data covering the period of a year, important questions can be answered.

Question	*Answer*
1. What is the frequency of medical care at public expense?	Compute the number of cases treated during the year per 1,000 eligible persons.
2. What is the frequency of specified types of medical care at public expense?	Compute the number of cases receiving specified types of care per 1,000 eligible persons.
3. What is the average amount of service provided at public expense?	Compute the number of such items as physicians' calls (home, office, day, night, hospital, etc.), dentists' visits, clinic visits, hospital days, drug prescriptions, and others per eligible person and per case of illness treated.
4. What is the total average cost of public medical care, inclusive and exclusive of administration?	Compute the total expenditures, inclusive and exclusive of those for administration, per eligible person and per case of illness treated.
5. What is the average cost of specified types of public medical care?	Compute the expenditures for each specified service per eligible person and per case of illness treated.
6. What is the proportional distribution of the various types of service and expenditures?	Determine the respective percentages.

Such statements, made annually, enable the people as well as their government to make a quantitative analysis of the work done at the taxpayers' expense, measure the state of the program as compared with preceding years, appraise the effectiveness of the various services as well as the total provisions, and plan for the future. Barring extraordinary events, the regular accounting makes it possible to estimate roughly the proportion of people seeking treatment, the

* In computing rates, service to the medically needy must be omitted as it cannot be related to a known unit of population.

average type and number of services demanded, the average cost of the total plan, and the proportion of the assistance budget needed to cover the operating costs of the public medical care program.

Cognizant of the great financial importance of public medical care and its growing social significance, some public agencies have begun to prepare and publish annual reports measuring up to scientific standards. The majority have continued to record a few financial figures only. Thus, surprisingly little is known about activities going on in thousands of localities throughout the country, as Louis S. Reed and Dean A. Clark have remarked.[98] The New Mexico Department of Public Welfare recently has published the results of a survey undertaken "to summarize the experience of the Department with medical care and the medical care program, and to secure as complete a picture as possible of the amount of unmet need for medical and health care among the open cases as of March 31, 1943." [99]

Illuminating as the few available reports are, they suffer from a fundamental defect. They describe agency activities rather than all tax-supported medical care within a political unit and, consequently, are of limited value to the appraisal of the over-all situation.

Experience as to Volume and Cost of Service

As accurate information is scant, no definite statement can be made about the frequency in which persons in need actually receive medical care at public expense.

That the demand for aid from public agencies is considerable even at a time when employment and earning possibilities are at a record high can be seen from the experience of Nassau County in the state of New York. In 1942 the welfare department of this political unit of approximately 400,000 people received 47,934 requests for medical care other than hospitalization. It approved 43,771 applications, including 19,118 for physicians' care, 1,848 for dental care, 25,526 for drugs, and 1,406 for miscellaneous items such as prosthetic devices and eyeglasses.[100]

The outstanding facts brought out by recent studies of general programs of public medical care are two. There is a striking inequality in the amount of care received by various categories of beneficiaries in the same locality and by the same groups in different communities. Furthermore, except for a few communities there is a wide spread between the service provided and the standards of adequate medical care set by experts, although high frequency and severity of illness are typical of the group usually accepted for public medical care. These findings reflect the great disparity in the present policies and procedures governing public medical care. The following figures from surveys conducted under the auspices of the United States Public Health Service before the war will serve to show pertinent details.[101]

In various localities of Minnesota and New York with relatively advanced medical care programs for beneficiaries of general assistance the average annual number of home calls ranged from 0.3 to 1.30 and that of office or clinic calls from 1 to 2 per eligible person. The average annual number of general hospital admissions ranged from 0.05 to 0.13, and that of days of hospitalization from 0.6 to 1.8 per eligible person.

In six medical care programs for recipients of old-age assistance the median number of home calls was 2.7, that of general hospital admissions 0.12, and that of days of general hospital hospital care 2.4 per eligible person.

In most of the localities the reported expenditures of welfare agencies for the general care of the sick in need are so much larger than all expenditures of public health agencies that one is reminded of the giant and the dwarf. The sums expended by the welfare departments in some counties account for the greater part of the total amount spent on health service by all public and private agencies.

With few exceptions, the published figures are not inclusive. Often the expenditures for the general care of the needy in governmental clinics, hospitals, and custodial institutions do not appear in the welfare agency reports, and the cost of administration are omitted in view of the difficulty of apportioning a proper share. Under such conditions it is not easy to compute and evaluate the total annual costs of the services provided by welfare departments. Where the data are complete they serve to analyze and appraise agency activities, but not more. The following results of studies of various local programs in a few states reveal many interesting facts.

In eight counties of Michigan the total average cost of "medical relief" in 1934 was estimated at $11.44 per person receiving direct relief. The figure includes expenses for physicians' care in the home, office, and hospital, hospital care, dental care, nursing care, eye care, drugs, surgical appliances, transportation, and administration.[102]

In two counties of Minnesota and in one city and one county in New

PROGRAMS FOR "PERSONS IN NEED" 149

York the cost of general medical care (excluding administration) for recipients of direct relief in 1939 ranged from $9.22 to $28.10 per eligible person. Table 1 gives details and also the distribution of costs by major types of service.[103]

TABLE 1

COST OF GENERAL MEDICAL CARE [a] FOR RECIPIENTS OF DIRECT RELIEF IN FOUR LOCALITIES, 1939

Average Cost per Eligible Person

Types of Care	County in Minnesota	County in Minnesota	City in New York	County in New York
Physicians' services	$3.74	$ 4.66	$ 3.89	$16.47
Dental care	0.60	1.15	0.64	0.81
General hospital care	2.60	5.27	9.50	8.61
Drugs	1.21	0.93	2.75	0.39
Other services	1.07	0.89	2.00	1.82
Total	$9.22	$12.90	$18.78	$28.10

[a] Excluding administration.

In one county in Virginia, one county in Minnesota, and one city and one county in New York the average expenditures for general medical care of recipients of old-age assistance ranged from as little as $4.70 per eligible person and year to as much as $31.25. (See Table 2.) Particularly noteworthy is the high proportion of the total spent on drugs.[104]

TABLE 2

COST OF GENERAL MEDICAL CARE [a] FOR RECIPIENTS OF OLD-AGE ASSISTANCE IN FOUR LOCALITIES

Average Cost per Eligible Person

	County in Virginia	County in Minnesota	City in New York	County in New York
Types of Care	1940–1941	1939	1939	1939
Physicians' services	$1.61	$ 2.90	$ 5.45	$ 8.66
Dental care	0.02	0.50	0.13	0.26
Nursing care	0.90	4.30	0.23	0.48
General hospital care	1.95	1.36	10.17	14.97
Drugs	0.07	4.79	4.25	6.11
Other services	0.15	0.61	0.67	0.77
Total	$4.70	$14.46	$20.90	$31.25

[a] Excluding administration.

The proportion of the total assistance expenditure spent on medical care varies widely. At present it is considerable where medically needy persons as well as recipients of public assistance are accepted and adequacy of service is emphasized. It is negligible where the eligibility standards are narrow and the provisions are limited to emergency service.

Outlays for medical care in general assistance agencies in 1940 accounted for 7 per cent of payments for relief in cash and kind.[105] In some instances a substantial proportion of the general assistance budget was absorbed by expenses for medical care. It amounted to 12 per cent in Freeborn County, Minnesota; 14 per cent in Chesterfield, Virginia; 22 per cent in Auburn, New York; and 43 per cent in all counties of North Dakota, to give a few examples only. It must be borne in mind that these figures show the extent to which assistance funds were used for a specific purpose, but not the part of the budget item that was spent on behalf of people receiving public assistance in general.

A multitude of agencies spend considerable amounts of tax funds either on general care of the needy sick or on special programs in which medical care accounts for a substantial fraction of the total expenses. Obviously, it would be of paramount importance to know the annual over-all cost of all tax-supported medical care in the community. To accomplish this all pertinent expenditures of all public agencies concerned must be assembled. The difficulties involved in such a project have proved so great that no reliable information has been presented.

Even if complete statistics could be brought together they would not conclusively answer the one question that is uppermost in the minds of many: What would be the average annual cost of adequate public medical care for persons in need? The obtainable cost figures are decisively influenced not only by the special, and quite different, needs of the various groups of people depending upon public aid but also by the policies followed in determining type, scope, amount, and period of service, accepting applicants for care at public expense, organizing professional services, and paying for the services of professional personnel and nongovernmental facilities. Moreover, it must be taken into account that nonprofit voluntary institutions and organizations are accorded the privilege of tax exemption.

· 5 ·

ADMINISTRATION OF PUBLIC MEDICAL CARE: ITS PRESENT FRAMEWORK

THE principles followed by public agencies in organizing the administration of selected types of public medical care have been discussed in the preceding chapters. To give that picture the necessary perspective, the broad policies adopted in building the framework of the administrative structure will be summarized briefly.

Over the years, three major trends of public policy have appeared. Power to administer direct service has been divided in a makeshift fashion between countless agencies of quite different types. Responsibility for budgeting and allocating public funds for the support of organized care of the sick has been distributed between a host of local, state, and Federal agencies which, often, are not identical with those responsible for direct administration. Authority to establish standards for public medical care has been given to a considerable number of different agencies, frequently to those having the power of the purse.

Traditionally, the establishment of each new type of service for the sick has carried with it the creation of a new administrative agency. The few known exceptions merely confirm the rule. Massachusetts, for instance, once had a single agency called the State Board of Health, Lunacy, and Charity—but only for the short period from 1877 to 1886.

What complicated the situation seriously was the tendency to carry the principle of division of administrative responsibility to the extreme. Each public agency which extended its functions to include provision of medical care set up a new bureau, office, division, or section for the administration of the new service, regardless of the fact that there were already a goodly number of units performing similar functions. This occurred because every agency, at each level of government, clung to the right of choosing and maintaining its own machinery for the administration of medical care no matter how inadequate it was. Besides, towns were jealous of the prerogatives which they yielded to the county, counties jealous of what they yielded to the state, and the states of what they yielded to the Federal government —to paraphrase H. Jackson Davis.[1]

Thus a vast number and infinite variety of official agencies now are concerned with administration of public medical care. From a functional point of view they may be classified in two broad categories: (1) agencies organized for the specific and sole purpose of administering health services, and (2) agencies vested with administrative authority for certain health services as part of a broader responsibility. Public health departments, hospital departments, and crippled children commissions exemplify the application of the principle of functional organization in different interpretations. The special units in various types of welfare agencies, labor departments, and educational authorities illustrate the second type of arrangement.

In itself, multiplicity of units administering direct service spells danger. Overlapping, if not duplication, of effort in some areas of activity and neglect in other areas equally essential might be hard to avoid. Disputes and friction among the agencies may impede the progress of the work, if not paralyze it. Direct waste of money by conflict of functions and indirect losses by delay and gaps in the treatment of the individual may ensue. Inconsistent and conflicting standards of service may be set. This potential danger has become real because public policy added a sin of omission to the sin of commission. It failed to bring about the badly needed clarification and reasonable demarcation of the powers and functions of the various agencies active in the same field, thereby missing the only chance of making the best of a bad situation. The inevitable result was diffusion of authority in the very fields that demand concentration of authority, and dissipation of function where unification was needed.

How serious the flaws in the administrative structure have become can be seen from the following list of widely used practices.

1. Public medical care for similar socio-economic groups in the same community is administered by different agencies. The type of disease or condition determines the distribution of responsibility. Such service as is essential to the effective campaign against communicable diseases ordinarily is under the jurisdiction of health departments. So is maternity care of wives and treatment of sick infants of enlisted men. Frequently, services for crippled children also are administered by health departments. On the other hand, medical care other than that provided under special programs falls mainly within the province of welfare departments of various types.

2. Identical types of care, such as home care or hospitalization, in

the same community are administered by a large variety of local, state, and Federal agencies. The determining factor is the socio-economic group to which the beneficiary belongs. The groups are numerous. They include recipients of general assistance (sometimes divided into employable and unemployable persons); recipients of old-age assistance, aid to the blind, and aid to dependent children; the medically needy not receiving other forms of public aid; and the veterans—to list only those large in number.

3. The same type of facility in different communities is administered by different agencies. No definite policy is followed in dividing administrative authority, except in the case of Federal hospitals. City, county, and state hospitals of the general type are under welfare departments; under special agencies such as hospital departments, departments of institutions, or hospital commissions; or—occasionally—under health departments. The state controlled tuberculosis hospitals are administered by health departments; by boards such as boards of control, boards of institutions, boards of charities and corrections; tuberculosis boards or commissions; and by departments of welfare in this order of frequency.[2] State activities which relate to mental deviations are concentrated within a single agency in only about one third of the states. Often they are administered by boards of control, hospital boards, and departments of institutions, and not infrequently by welfare departments. In addition, health departments, boards or commissions of mental hygiene, state universities, and other agencies exercise administrative functions in this field.[3]

4. The same type of special program in different political units is administered by different agencies. A typical case in point are the crippled children's programs. In 1942 they were administered by health departments in twenty-nine instances, welfare departments in ten instances, educational authorities in five instances, special commissions in five instances, and state universities in three instances.[4]

To these examples of administrative confusion many more could be added without exhausting the topic.[5] But they suffice to explain why all observers are agreed on one point: the house urgently needs rebuilding from the bottom up.

The concepts on distribution of financial responsibility for public medical care have changed markedly in recent times. It has been recognized that small political units of government are unsuited to the task of fully supporting adequate institutions and services, although they may be useful for administration of direct service. In general, the obligation to establish facilities which are beyond the financial capacity of small units has been shifted to large subdivisions of the state or the state itself. Responsibility for payment of services rendered through these facilities to persons eligible for public aid, if not assumed by the state, has been divided between town and county, town or city and state, or county and state. In a growing number of instances, the principle of cost sharing by various political units also has been applied to programs of medical care. Gradually, at different rates of speed and to widely varying extents, state-local cooperation is superseding isolated local efforts.

A partnership between localities and the state has been generally established for the advancement of public health work and greatly contributed to the improvement of treatment services for persons with certain diseases, defects, or conditions. It has been organized for the operation of assistance programs for dependent children, the blind, and the old, thereby somewhat facilitating the support of the general medical care of these groups. In a few states only has it been extended to programs of general assistance and thus begun to influence the development of more adequate medical care for the needy not covered by special programs.

Apart from the disparity in basic policy of administrative organization, another shortcoming has retarded the progress of public medical care. Some states raise uniform taxes on a state-wide basis, thus pooling the resources of wealthier and poorer areas. Other states differentiate the tax rate according to localities, with the result that the funds available for poorer districts remain insufficient.

The increased use and marked improvement of the time-tested device of state-local cooperation in financing medical care is largely due to the development of systematic Federal-state cooperation following the adoption of the Social Security Act of 1935. Federal grants-in-aid to the states for the support of health services have come to play a notable role in American health policy. Of particular significance is the steady and rapid increase in allocations of tax money for fields of activity in which provision of adequate treatment is of paramount importance. The Federal grants to the states for the control of venereal diseases have increased from $3,000,000 in 1938–39 to $8,750,000 in 1941–42, and those for the operation of crippled children's programs from $2,850,000 in 1936–37 to $3,870,000 in 1941–42.

Originally, the allotment of Federal funds was made on the basis of a matching requirement, that is, the Federal government disbursed funds only to states spending money for designated purposes and only in an amount equal to that of approved state expenditures. Soon the fifty-fifty formula proved to be inappropriate. States with meager resources of their own could obtain but small amounts of supplementary funds although they needed aid badly. Those with ample tax income were benefited substantially although their needs were less pressing. To remedy this situation, the principle of equalization was incorporated into the statutes governing the allotment of Federal grants-in-aid. At present the actual requirements of each state as well as the amount of state funds available for matching are taken into consideration in determining the annual allocations of Federal funds to the states.

Only a few areas of public health activities were singled out for preferential development through joint support from the Federal government and the states. Many special programs which depend for their efficacy on provision of adequate medical care have not received the attention they deserve and, consequently, remained in a state of infancy.

Besides selected public health services only the assistance programs of the states for the old, blind, and dependent children are subsidized by the Federal government under the terms of the Social Security Act. The Federal share is fixed at half of the assistance payments up to a monthly maximum of $40 in old-age assistance and aid to the blind, and at $18 for the first child and $12 for each additional child receiving aid for dependent children.

Because of the multitude of agencies involved and the multiplicity of schedules used in allocating funds, the present system of administering funds for public medical care is unwieldy and wasteful. An army of clerks is required to figure out "who pays for whom, for what, and how much," and another army of auditors is needed to check the accuracy of the payments.

With the establishment of partnerships between local, state, and Federal governments it has become possible to better the quality of facilities, personnel, and services provided at public expense and to promote adequacy as well as uniformity of tax-supported programs for the sick. As cooperation between the three governments is limited to selected programs, standardization of public medical care has made progress only in some special fields rather than in general.

The ways and means by which improvements in organized care of the sick actually are attained are many and varied. Nation-wide as well as state-wide planning—including the establishment of standards for facilities, personnel, services, and administrative organization—are receiving increasing attention. Professional direction of medical care facilities and programs for the treatment of the sick is slowly but steadily taking the place of lay direction. Health departments, with few exceptions, now are headed by physicians appointed on the basis of merit, unlike some decades ago when business background or political activity were regarded as proper qualifications. In contrast, many other agencies administering medical care employ no medical administrators. Professional advice through committees representing the various groups concerned is secured more frequently. Technical direction and supervision of services through competent members of the various health professions are in process of development.

The more the importance of standardization of public medical care is recognized, the more the lack of trained medical administrators makes itself felt. The medical colleges and public health schools in the United States, like those in many other countries in past years, have been slow to adjust their plans of instruction to new needs and new professional opportunities.

As history shows, the forces representing organized care of the sick and the forces representing public health not only marched but also fought separately in the past. They still do. Public policy thus neglects the primary rule of grand strategy—to beat the enemy by joint operation. In line with the doctrine of separate action the administration of public medical care has been set up apart from the administration of preventive services emphasizing diagnosis and health education. This practice has been abandoned only in a few sectors of the vast battlefield in which the fight against disease, defect, and human suffering is waged. The question, then, may well be raised whether there is any justification for the continuation of such administrative organization, admittedly anything but conducive to the efficacy of health service.

In some fields public facilities and programs of medical care have slowly but steadily superseded nongovernmental institutions and services. In other fields voluntary groups have continued to occupy a dominant position. The cold hard fact is that the activities of both groups have long been carried out without any coordination and only recently have been somewhat harmonized in a few areas of work. Is it a hopeless undertaking to design an administrative structure favoring integration of closely related parts?

> We might as well require a man to wear still the coat which fitted him when a boy as civilized society to remain ever under the regimen of their barbarous ancestors.—THOMAS JEFFERSON

Part II: Directed Growth

· 6 ·

PLANNING FOR MEDICAL CARE

ANY country aspiring to "a genuine and rational economy of human resources and values" [1] sooner or later will have to decide on both the broad objectives of its future health policy and the basic methods of organizing and financing adequate services. Wherever a broad program is visualized—and what enlightened nation would dare evade such a task—it implies over-all planning of health service in the widest sense of the term and, thus, planning for medical care.

Planning for medical care is inevitable. The rise of scientific medicine, with specialization becoming a characteristic feature, has greatly increased available knowledge and skill, scientific and technical. Medical care has become more efficient but also more complex and more expensive. Profound economic and social changes have had a strong bearing on the need, demand, and individual ability to pay for all the services modern medicine has to offer, with the result that a gap has been widening between medical science and practice. The magnitude and seriousness of the problem of illness from the social and economic viewpoints have led to the realization that adjustments are necessary in the interest of all: patients, professions, institutions, and society as a whole.

Such readjustments are beyond the power of the individual and of any single group to achieve. They cannot be brought about by haphazard development of multiple separate programs, one set designed for the control of a variety of diseases and another set for the care of a variety of population groups. They cannot be attained by keeping personal services for the prevention of illness and promotion of good health at arm's length from those for the treatment of the sick. They cannot be accomplished by disarticulated forces, one representing public and the other voluntary efforts.

In general, planning for medical care aims at the organization of those facilities and services which are necessary to prevent, cure, and mitigate illness and to reduce, if not prevent, disability, economic insecurity, and dependency. Specifically, it endeavors to make better what is already good and eliminate, once and for all, what is bad in the available services; fill gaps in the existing community health programs; and eliminate duplication, overlapping, and waste of effort. It tries to promote efficient and economical utilization of financial resources, public and private; coordinate and increase the efficacy of separate facilities, services, and agencies; avoid failure in lines too strongly specialized; strengthen and balance the whole program; and, ultimately, achieve quantitative and qualitative adequacy of all facilities and services.

The attainment of these objectives requires planning for (1) medical care facilities serving the community; (2) organized professional services; (3) methods of payment for both the establishment of necessary facilities and the services rendered by institutions and health professions; and (4) administrative procedures to assure early diagnosis, early, prompt, and thorough treatment, high standards of service, and continuity and consistency of care.

These are all parts of an integral whole. They cannot be separated without injuring all. To maintain the best facilities without organizing the payment for their use is like inviting people to enter a locked house without giving them the key. "To urge postponement of more adequate financing arrangements on the grounds that quality of service is primary and that payment is secondary is like saying that the quality of construction of a house is primary and the financing and mortgage arrangements are secondary." [2] To establish organized medical care without setting up a sound administration for it is like seeding without watering and weeding.

Standing alone, even the best medical care program cannot solve the multitude of problems arising out of sickness, injury, and maternity. It must rest on the firm foundation of services minimizing the risk of illness due to environmental conditions, and of systematic education in personal hygiene, physical fitness, and the full and discriminating use of available services. It must be supported by a program of economic security in general and of protection against the economic consequences of temporary and permanent disability in particular. It must be strengthened by close cooperation with social work.

To meet the individual's requirements as well as the community's need for adequate, humane, and economical service, a medical care program must be broad in scope and well balanced. It must provide for all services needed by the apparently healthy, acutely sick, convalescent, and chronically ill, including care at the home, office, clinic, general hospital, special hospital, and custodial institution, in the amount and for the period required. It must apply to sickness, defect, injury, and maternity.

Components of an adequate program of medical care are:

1. Physicians' service, including general practitioners and specialists
2. Dental service, including dentists and dental hygienists
3. Nursing service, including institutional and public health nurses, nurse-midwives, nurses' aides, and visiting housekeepers
4. Medical social service, including case workers and persons engaged in organization and administration of health service
5. Diagnostic laboratory and roentgenological services
6. Supply of drugs, diets, and appliances
7. Special treatment services, such as physical therapy and roentgen and radium therapy
8. Hospitalization in general and special hospitals, including convalescent homes and hospitals for the chronically ill
9. Custodial care in institutions
10. Ambulance service

PLANNING FOR HOSPITALS AND RELATED FACILITIES

A well-organized system of adequate hospitals and related medical care facilities is basic to social progress as well as to individual welfare. It requires for its development a master plan that clearly defines the basic policy as to the establishment, improvement, and operation of both governmental and nongovernmental facilities. Decisions are necessary on the following points:

I. Degree of concentration of hospital beds in large units
II. Degree of specialization of hospitals
III. Quantitative standards for the various types of hospitals and related facilities
IV. Qualitative standards for the various types of hospitals and related facilities

V. Responsibility for the provision of hospitals and related facilities
VI. Function of the general hospital in the community health program
VII. Functional coordination of general and special hospitals
VIII. Method of organizing hospital service
IX. Function of the medical center in the community health program

I. There are weighty reasons for the concentration of beds in a limited number of large hospitals serving geographical areas and against continued building of numerous few-bed facilities for service to small political units.

Only hospitals of sufficient size can organize a competent professional staff including representatives of the major specialties. Only they can afford and fully utilize the elaborate and costly equipment necessary for good medical care and still operate comparatively economically through spreading the costs of the services, including the fixed charges, among the large number of patients treated. What is not less important, they offer great opportunities for research as well as for professional education and postgraduate training of various groups. With the development of rapid transportation, with motor-car and airplane constantly reducing the obstacles of space and time, the revision of the "small hospital" policy, justified in the horse and buggy age, is becoming feasible.

There are two important arguments against the elimination of the small facility. The neighborhood hospital, even if it is an infirmary in fact, might be of great importance to the local physicians. Without association with a medical care facility, the neighborhood doctors might find it next to impossible to carry out such professional work as they are competent to do and maintain certain standards of practice. Small institutions are necessary for the care of bedridden patients with minor illnesses, if the main hospitals are to be utilized effectively and economically. They may be valuable in case of emergencies.

What, then, is a "small" hospital? Experts in various countries differ little in their answers to this question. In the United States the official statistics classify as very small the hospitals with less than 25 beds and as small those having 25 to 49 beds. In Sweden facilities with less than about 70 beds, in Germany those with less than 50 beds, and in some French cities those with less than 60 beds are regarded as small. It is noteworthy that in Sweden a facility with less than 30 beds is called a "cottage hospital" and designated only for the care of minor illnesses and emergencies.

The definition of a "large" hospital is much debated. The reports of the United States Bureau of the Census distinguish between medium-sized hospitals having 50 to 99 beds and large hospitals with a capacity of 100 beds and more. Many experts believe that only facilities of 200 beds and more should be termed "large."

What is the optimum capacity for general and various types of special hospitals? Do general hospitals of 400 or 600 beds offer advantages over those with more than 1,000 beds as is claimed by some students of the subject? Are mental hospitals of 1,500 beds preferable to city-like facilities accommodating 6,000 patients? Is a tuberculosis hospital of 200 to 400 beds superior to one of 1,000 beds? In short, how far can the principle of concentration of beds be carried without creating difficulties in operating and administering the institution and without hindering its easy adaptation to new conditions? These are still open questions. Bigness as such does not necessarily spell adequacy, economy, and convenience of service. The relative merits of hospitals of various size require careful study before definitive decisions about the future direction of hospital policy are made.

II. Each advance in scientific medicine and therapeutic methods necessarily involves adjustments in the hospital program. Not infrequently, it is immediately followed by proposals for the construction of a new type of special facility. If such requests were met without an over-all plan for the building and operation of all types of hospitals, the result would be an uncoordinated mass of numerous facilities with limited functions. It would become a mere aggregation of parts. Scientific and technological progress, on the other hand, may make superfluous many a separate facility deemed necessary before. The issue, then, is this: Should the general hospital be enlarged and equipped with new special divisions as need and opportunity arise or should the building of separate specialized facilities be encouraged?

As ample experience has shown, the general hospital—if well organized, well equipped, properly staffed, and intelligently operated—can take over many of the functions traditionally carried out by separate units. This is particularly true of the care of patients with infectious diseases, including venereal diseases and certain stages of tuberculosis, and—within limits—of the treatment of patients with certain mental deviations. A goodly number of the existing small hospitals which concentrate on a single disease or group of diseases could be gradually eliminated. New construction of separate communicable disease hospitals appears no longer justified except in metropolitan areas and large sea and air ports, and for the special purpose of detaining patients who cannot be left at large.

On the other hand, certain special hospitals and related institutions are indispensable to meet the medical, socio-economic, and psychological requirements of clearly definable groups of patients as well as the community's need for adequate, humane, and economical service. In addition, they are valuable as research and teaching centers.

The sick requiring the services of special hospitals may be classified in three broad categories. In the first group belong mainly patients in a certain stage of mental illness, tuberculosis, crippling condition, heart disease, and rheumatic condition, although other diseases or disease groups may be added to the list when indicated. The second group comprises patients recovering progressively from acute or chronic illness after disappearance of serious disability, and persons with minor illnesses and borderline conditions not requiring the services of a general or special hospital. A third group is represented by patients considerably disabled by chronic physical illness, and this is certain to grow appreciably with the increase in the average length of life. In all three groups the stage of illness rather than the type of disease is one of the major factors determining the individual's need for care in a special facility.

From the community point of view the cost of special hospitals and related medical care facilities deserve special consideration. Although no generalizations are possible a few details are worth mentioning. Adequate facilities for convalescent care can be built at less than one half and operated at about one half to two thirds of the cost required for a general hospital designed for the acutely sick. Adequate chronic hospitals cost less to construct and maintain than general hospitals. The economies attainable vary a good deal depending upon the type of facility, its organization as an independent unit or part of a general hospital, and its utilization for certain patients. They may be comparatively small or may reach substantial proportions, such as one half of the building costs and three fifths of the operating costs of hospitals for the acutely sick.

III. The quantitative standards at present recommended in the United States for various types of hospitals have been referred to in

Chapter Two. How many hospital beds per unit of population are necessary is hard to determine. Before making a decision many and diverse factors must be weighed as to their potential effect on both the need and demand for hospitalization. These factors are as follows:

A. Socio-economic factors
 1. Size, sex and age distribution, and probable development of the population residing in the "hospital area," with due consideration to seasonal influx of temporary residents and frequency of transients
 2. Character of the area, that is, whether predominantly urban or rural; number and size of towns located in rural districts and of suburban developments and rural parts in urban areas; probable trends
 3. Types of occupation prevailing in the hospital area, and especially type and frequency of industries
 4. Housing conditions
 5. Economic conditions and, in particular, financial resources available for (*a*) the establishment of adequate hospitals and (*b*) the payment of hospital care
 6. Educational level and habits and customs of the population
 7. Transportation facilities

B. Health conditions
 1. Frequency of births
 2. Type, frequency, and severity of physical and mental diseases and defects and of injuries
 3. Mortality, by major causes of death

C. Availability of services other than hospital care
 1. Type, number, distribution, and utilization of services designed for case-finding, early diagnosis, health guidance and follow-up; application of such services as vaccination and immunization
 2. Number, distribution, and utilization of treatment clinics, visiting nurse services, plans providing home and office care, and specialized services such as family care of mentally ill persons

D. Number and attitude of the practicing physicians toward hospitalization
 1. Number of physicians in relation to the population, and especially number of such specialists as surgeons and obstetricians
 2. Prevailing attitude in regard to use of hospitals, in particular

for deliveries, care of common communicable diseases, and treatment of mental deviations
E. Organized payment for hospitalization
  1. Policies and procedures in providing care at public expense
  2. Voluntary and compulsory insurance plans covering hospitalization in case of maternity, sickness, and injury

In view of the great disparity in the conditions prevailing in different sections of the same country, it seems advisable for practical purposes to establish standard bed rates, by type of hospitals, for sections of the country rather than for the country as a whole. Such indices must be revised at regular intervals. New developments, in particular advances in scientific medicine, expansion of preventive health services, large-scale organization of payment for hospitalization, and marked changes in the composition of the population, may either increase or decrease the need for hospital service. They may intensify or reduce the demand for such type of care.

IV. To prevent the building and operation of substandard facilities for the care of the sick, the general adoption of the following policies appears necessary:
  1. Formulation and revision, when indicated, of the minimum requirements to be met by any medical care facility, and of standards for institutions to be approved as hospitals. Clear definition of the conditions to be satisfied for each type of institution, with emphasis on such questions as grounds and buildings, equipment, professional staff, and administrative organization
  2. Licensing of all governmental and nongovernmental facilities designated for the care of the sick, the license to be issued for either an "infirmary" or a "hospital," as the case may be (The American Hospital Association has prepared a "model law".)
  3. Regular inspection and rating of all medical care facilities

V. If there is to be any effective planning for hospitals the problem of responsibility for their provision must be settled.

It may be proposed to abandon the voluntary system, whether it is devoted to the common good or to the pursuit of gain, and declare support of hospitals a right and a duty of government. Opponents to such "socialization of hospitals" in the strict sense of the word may insist that public policy should not "deny scope and opportunity in one of the most appealing fields to the expression and practice of freely accorded individual benevolence." [3] It should do everything to preserve the voluntary hospital system in its vigor and volume. Acceptance of this tenet implies obligations for both governmental agencies and nongovernmental groups interested in the development and support of hospitals. Obviously there is little justification for the continued existence of three sets of hospitals—governmental, nonprofit voluntary, and proprietary—if the result is wasteful duplication of accommodation, equipment, and services in one area and lack or scarcity of hospitals in others. What appears to be necessary is (1) coordination of public and private resources for the building of new hospitals and expansion and improvement of existing ones according to proved community needs; (2) division of labor between governmental and nongovernmental hospitals on the basis of the functions they are best equipped to perform; and (3) coordination among hospitals in the appointment of their medical staffs, in particular certain specialists. This will require some sacrifices on the part of voluntary groups. But, to quote the Hospital Council of Greater New York, "The continued usefulness of the voluntary hospitals, as institutions free to pioneer and lead in the development of hospital care, in medical research, and in the training of physicians and nurses, will depend not on a great number of these hospitals receiving extensive governmental support and supervision, but on the sound operation of a smaller number so competently organized, staffed, equipped and financed by voluntary leadership that they render an outstanding service to the community." [4]

VI. Prior to any decision about the function of the general hospital a much disputed problem must be settled—do hospitals practice medicine? The Board of Trustees of the American Hospital Association has given the following answer which speaks for itself:

1. The primary obligation of the hospital is to provide all the services necessary for the diagnosis, treatment and rehabilitation of the patient.
2. Provision of medical services in hospitals is part of the responsibility of the hospital, and is consistent with the rights, privileges, and obligations of hospital staff physicians under their medical licensure. The performance of diagnostic and therapeutic procedures by staff members constitutes the practice of medicine *in* hospitals. It is not the practice of medicine *by* hospitals.
3. The employment of a physician by a hospital is consistent with law and with professional ethics and does not imply that the hospital is engaged in the practice of medicine.

4. The financial arrangement between a hospital and a physician is not a determining factor in the ethics or legality of medical practice in hospitals.[5]

Opinions about the part to be played by the general hospital in the future community health program differ sharply.

One group of experts hold that the general hospital should be developed into the center for organized care of the sick by integration of hospital service, clinic service, and home care. They want to broaden the application of a principle expressed in the following words: "Hospitals should be organized and conducted primarily for the purpose of providing facilities where the sick and the injured of the community may be given scientific and ethical medical care." [6] Extension of hospital service as suggested implies that governmental as well as nonprofit voluntary hospitals accept any patient rather than selected groups in the community. To make this policy possible, statutes preventing city, county, and state hospitals from admitting persons other than the indigent should be abolished. Nonprofit voluntary hospitals meeting official standards should be fully utilized and adequately compensated by public agencies.

A second school of thought visualizes a much wider function for the general hospital. As Michael M. Davis said: "The hospital should be the physical and the organizational center through which physicians and the allied professions would supply all forms of medical service to the community." [7] It would serve not only the sick by providing and organizing all the services necessary for diagnosis, treatment, care, and rehabilitation, but also the healthy by carrying out preventive health work. The hospital would be the base from which the health professions would conduct their practice. This idea assumes the development of group practice of medicine, as recommended by the majority of the Committee on the Costs of Medical Care.[8] Pertinent details will be discussed in the subsequent section on Planning for Organization of Professional Services.

To what extent the hospital can be utilized effectively for preventive as well as therapeutic services depends not only on the organization of medical practice but also on the distribution of hospital facilities in the future. If concentration of beds in a small number of main hospitals and specialization of large facilities are emphasized as they should be, one conclusion is inescapable: decentralized facilities must be provided for routine services. District medical centers will have to be established wherever practicable, and they would perform a good many of the functions otherwise assigned to the main hospital.

VII. General and special hospitals, nongovernmental as well as governmental, should be functionally coordinated through understandings among all groups concerned. Such cooperation, apart from promoting research and teaching, offers tangible and immediate advantages to the operation of medical care programs. The sick can be directly admitted or be promptly transferred to the facility best suited to their needs. The period of stay in the hospital with highly organized diagnostic and treatment service and specialized professional personnel can be shortened. Beds in various types of facilities can be utilized properly. Thus, considerable savings can be achieved for all: the patients, the organization or agency paying for their care, and the community anxious to develop and support adequate institutional facilities at reasonable cost.

VIII. Detailed proposals for revision of the hospital policy have been offered by leading experts and representative groups in various countries. All recommend regional organization of hospital services, the logical corollary to the principles of concentration and differentiation of facilities. This idea is not new. In many countries it has long guided public policy in organizing the services of specialized hospitals, particularly those for mental and tuberculous patients. In a few countries it has been applied to general hospitals. The Dominion of New Zealand, for instance, is divided into forty-two hospital districts, each under the control of a hospital board.

In France it was mainly M. Sarraz-Bournet who on many occasions suggested planning hospitals on the basis of large areas, the *départements*. In 1932 he stated his ideas as follows: (1) one main well-equipped general hospital *(hôpital de grand rattachement)* as the center for all organized care of the sick, with several less completely equipped hospitals *(hôpitaux de rattachement)* distributed over the area; (2) discontinuation of the use of facilities with fewer than 50 beds as general hospitals, prohibition of new construction of such units, and utilization of existing buildings as emergency stations *(postes de secours)* or institutions for the old, infirm, or chronically sick; and (3) provision of special hospitals on a regional basis.[9]

In Great Britain regional organization of voluntary hospitals was suggested in the report of the Voluntary Hospitals Committee as long ago as 1921. "For several years the Department of Health for Scotland has advocated joint action for hospital purposes by local authorities and voluntary bodies over wide regions with teaching centres at their bases. The British Medical Association has urged the grouping of hospitals round a central or base hospital, while the Voluntary Hospitals Commission, set up by the British Hospitals Association in 1935, recommended the division of the country into hospital regions with the formation in each region of an Advisory Council, and the formation of a Central Council, also advisory, to correlate the work of the regions." [10] Regionalization has been greatly stimulated by the establishment, in 1939, of the Nuffield Provincial Hospitals Trust and accelerated by the impact of the war. In 1942 the Medical Planning Commission of the British Medical Association as well as an independent group of anonymous physicians [11] included in their recommendations for the future organization of medical care the tenet that the region or subregion should be the unit of the hospital service. The Government, in 1944, not only stated that "for the future hospital service, it will be essential to obtain larger local areas than at present, both for planning and administration" but also made definite proposals for the attainment of this principle.[12]

In Australia the National Health and Medical Research Council suggested applying the principle of regional organization throughout the populated sections of the country. "In the metropolitan areas and in a few of the larger cities there should be, in addition to the central hospitals, a ring of suburban consultation centres for primary consultations and casualty treatment and of small hospitals for minor cases. These local centres and hospitals would be staffed by local medical men and would relieve the central hospitals, which should be kept for serious and specialist cases." [13]

IX. Students of the subject are agreed that a unified service for the healthy and the sick is necessary from the point of view of the people to be served, the health professions, the medical care facilities, and the community at large. As Kendall Emerson remarked: "The time is over-ripe . . . to stop talking about curative and preventive medicine, to use instead the designation 'medical care,' whether that care is furnished to the absolutely healthy, the mildly indisposed, the acutely ill, or the chronic invalid." [14]

How can the ideal of unified medical care be realized? Should medical centers be established for inclusive service to the community? If so, how should they be built, equipped, staffed, supported, administered, and functionally related to other facilities and services? These questions are inextricably bound to the larger problems of organizing and paying for professional services. These will be discussed in subsequent sections.

PLANNING FOR ORGANIZATION OF PROFESSIONAL SERVICES

Professional services constituting an integral part of a well-rounded and well-balanced health program for the community may be organized on the basis of individual practice, group practice, or both side by side. Whatever the method of organization, every effort must be made to assure competence, sufficient number, and reasonable distribution of the members of the various health professions. The essential thing is to formulate an over-all plan outlining the basic policy to be pursued and its application under various conditions.

The activities of the members of the various professional groups should be restricted to the bounds of their competence. Axiomatic as this principle is, it is hard to attain, particularly in the case of physicians. The license to practice medicine is generic. It gives the holder the right to engage in any or all branches of medicine. There is no requirement of special preparation for those who want to practice a specialty. However, the medical profession voluntarily has established standards for certification as a specialist. In addition, a growing number of hospitals have come to set strict conditions for admission to and work on their staffs.

The problem, then, is to apply generally and enforce by appropriate administrative procedures principles that are already introduced but not yet in common use. Any physician licensed to practice medicine should be admitted to the program, but the scope of his activities should be determined on the basis of his professional education and special experience and confined to the fields of his demonstrated competence. If hospitals are opened to all physicians who are licensed under the laws of the state to practice medicine in the hospital area, "regulations must be established which will limit the professional privileges of each according to his training and proficiency, so that no man may be permitted to attempt tasks beyond his capacity." [15] The stricter this principle is enforced by hospital authorities the smaller the danger of deterioration of standards.

Standards for the number of professional personnel needed to give adequate medical care to a unit of population are useful as general guides. But they must be determined under due consideration of both the need and demand for good medical care, and be revised at regular intervals to be suited to conditions prevailing at a given time.

In determining ratios for physicians, dentists, pharmacists, visiting nurses, medical social workers, and other groups, a large number and variety of factors must be taken into account. They include (1) socio-economic conditions; (2) habits and attitudes of the people; (3) health conditions; (4) type and number of medical care facilities; (5) type and number of organized programs of medical care; (6) type and extent of health and welfare activities, both governmental and nongovernmental; and (7) method of organization of professional services.

In their classical study *The Fundamentals of Good Medical Care*, Roger I. Lee and Lewis W. Jones have estimated the number of various services needed to supply good medical care.[16] Similar studies, conducted on a broader basis and repeated from time to time, will be of great value in arriving at sound decisions on standard figures for the provision of professional personnel.

Of particular importance to planning for the immediate future is the problem of demand for medical care. As a puzzled physician in a small town once wrote in a letter: "The trouble is that the people ask too much nowadays. The pioneers were satisfied if they could have a doctor only at most critical illnesses. . . . People have come to expect of medical service not merely care in time of acute or serious illness; they have come to expect that it will prevent disease, promote health, and enlarge life." Education in general and health education in particular create and intensify demand for medical care. Establishment of a broad health program, or expansion and improvement of existing services, including organized payment for the use of facilities and professional services, enable large numbers of people to translate their desire for medical care into effective demand. Thus, in the initial stage, the services of a newly installed or extended and improved program will be sought extensively, some more than others. In a later stage, the demand is likely to fall off, and the average period for which certain services such as general hospital care, have to be provided can be expected to decline.

Scientific advances, resulting in the introduction of new preventive, diagnostic, or therapeutic methods, and improvements in public health policy and practices may result in a temporary rise in demand for certain professional services but, ultimately, will in many instances reduce the need for them.

What makes the calculation of adequate ratios particularly difficult is the fact that it is humanly impossible to draw a satisfactory dividing line between the scientifically necessary and the subjectively desirable. Some patients are "doctor-conscious." They turn automatically to the physician for the treatment of minor ailments or disturbances or merely in search of sympathy and attention. To brand such demands as "abuse" appears contrary to the avowed aims of modern medicine. If the physician is to be the counselor of the healthy and the helper of the sick, if true psychosomatic medicine is to be practiced, if early diagnosis and treatment are to be encouraged —then all but plainly unwarranted demands of the patients must be satisfied. These demands are clearly beyond the bounds of any general statistical estimate. They will have to be evaluated locally on the basis of observation. The only—rather limited—experience available at present is gained from the operation of group practice plans for self-supporting persons in the middle and lower income brackets. It appears that one full-time physician for every 1,000 to 1,200 persons would be needed to provide fairly complete medical care. This figure does not include service to patients in special facilities, such as mental and tuberculosis hospitals.

The evil of utterly uneven distribution of health personnel, with wealthy sections and urban areas oversupplied and poorer sections and rural areas sadly undersupplied, is not incurable. What is necessary to remedy the situation, is the determination to apply principles of action that have already proved their value. They are: (1) construction of good medical care facilities where needed, in particular in rural areas; (2) organization of payment for health service so that professional persons are assured of a satisfactory income whether they practice in a metropolis or a small town; (3) establishment of central registers, primarily for physicians and dentists, which list vacant practices as well as localities desiring a physician or dentist and submitting necessary information including evidence of need; (4) limitation of the number of patients a physician or dentist may accept under a designated program; (5) financial assistance to professional persons willing to move to a locality with established need; and (6) scholarships for students of medicine, dentistry, nursing, and social work who later will stay a stated number of years in rural areas.

However, one point cannot be emphasized too strongly. Efforts to bring about a better distribution of health personnel will be seriously impeded unless nation-wide licenses are substituted for state licenses.

Group Practice

Group practice, already systematically carried forward in a few countries, is under serious consideration for introduction in a score of countries making plans for the improvement of medical care. Its principles and its development in the United States have been discussed in Chapter Three. To clarify such points as are of particular importance to future planning, selected proposals for the introduction of group practice will be reviewed briefly.

In the United States the Committee on the Costs of Medical Care made history by proposing a new approach to a satisfactory medical service. The committee consisted of fifty members representing the fields of private practice, public health, medical institutions and special interests, the social sciences, and the general public. In 1932 these experts made public the valuable results of a five-year program of fact finding. A majority placed at the head of five recommendations the tenet "that medical service, both preventive and therapeutic, should be furnished largely by organized groups of physicians, dentists, nurses, pharmacists, and other associated personnel. Such groups should be organized, preferably around a hospital, for rendering complete home, office, and hospital care. The form of organization should encourage the maintenance of high standards and the development or preservation of a personal relation between patient and physician."

Opposition to this proposal was registered by a minority group on the following grounds: "(1) It [the medical center plan] would establish a medical hierarchy in every community to dictate who might practice medicine there. This is inherent in the plan since any new member of the center must be chosen either by the chief or by a small staff. (2) It would be impossible to prevent competition among the many such centers necessary for large cities; cost would inevitably be increased by the organization necessary to assign patients to the various centers. This would add to the evils of medical dictatorship those of a new bureau in the local government with its attendant cost. (3) Continuous personal relationship of physician and patient would be difficult if not impossible under such conditions." [17] An editorial in the *Journal of the American Medical Association* had this to say: "The alignment is clear—on the one side the forces representing the great foundations, public health officialdom, social theory— even socialism and communism inciting to revolution; on the other side the organized medical profession of the country urging an orderly evolution." [18]

Since that time the idea of group practice has been promoted primarily by the Committee of Physicians for the Improvement of Medical Care (John P. Peters, Secretary), organized in 1937 to protect and advance the quality of medical care in all programs that might be instituted.[19] The establishment of sound group practice schemes has been furthered by voluntary organizations such as the Committee on Research in Medical Economics (Michael M. Davis, Chairman) and the Medical Administration Service (Kingsley Roberts, Director). No official action has been taken, nor is the term group practice mentioned in the Wagner-Murray-Dingell Bill, introduced in Congress on May 24, 1943.

In Great Britain, as early as 1920, the government-appointed Dawson Committee recommended the use of regional centers for both medical practice and public health work, thereby officially endorsing suggestions repeatedly offered before by private groups.[20] In the early forties two medical organizations went on record in favor of group practice.

The Medical Planning Commission, established by the British Medical Association in August, 1940, stated that "group or cooperative general practice is desirable, though some variation of the organization would be necessary in sparsely populated areas" and offered a detailed plan of a "Model Health Centre." The building and equipment of the center would be provided or approved by the regional authority in charge of the comprehensive medical service. Its medical staff "would consist of a number of principals and assistants" and "each principal would have his own list of persons who select him. . . . Health visitors and district nurses, like midwives, would be based on the centre, and they would assist in all the work of the centre." The service would be available to everybody. It would be "preventive and educational, as well as curative," include general medical care at the center and in the home of the patient, but exclude specialists' services provided "at special clinics with specialist staffs. . . . The medical staff as a whole would assume responsibility for the ante-natal, post-natal, infant welfare, and school medical work which is at present rendered by the medical staff of local authorities." [21]

Medical Planning Research, an organization of four hundred British physicians in the younger age groups, offered similar proposals and stressed that "the centre should encourage an emphasis on health rather than sickness in the community it serves." After careful consideration of all sides of the problem, the authors of the plan arrived at this conclusion: "We consider that the only serious risk of the health centre system is that it may lead to bickering and quarreling among the home doctors [that is, the family doctors or general practitioners] working there. Nevertheless, the advantages, both to patients and staff, which it offers, greatly outweigh this risk. . . . With a certain amount of good will we see no reason why the rivalry inside the health centre should not be confined to healthy and stimulating competition." [22]

The British Medical Association in 1943 resolved: "That there should be initiated, by arrangement and agreement between the Government and the profession, organized experiments in methods of practice, such as group practice, including health centres of different kinds, which should extend to the general practitioner hospital units attached to general hospitals." [23]

The British government in 1944 acknowledged that " 'grouped' practices . . . must have a high place in the planning of the new service" [the National Health Service] and announced that the group idea would be placed "in the forefront of their plans in order that there may be a full trial on a large scale of the working of arrangements of this kind. . . . The new service shall be based on a combination of grouped practice and of separate practice side by side." [24]

In Australia the National Health and Medical Research Council —a body representing departments of health, both commonwealth and state, universities having medical schools, the Colleges of Physicians and of Surgeons, and the Federal Council of the British Medical Association in Australia—proposed introduction of group practice and establishment of a system of "consultation centres."

"The basic idea of the consultation centre is that every sick person who is reasonably mobile and who does not need treatment at a hospital, should be treated at the consultation centre instead of at his home." These facilities would "take over [from the hospitals] and return to the general practitioner that large mass of general practice now dealt with at hospitals as out-patient practice." [25]

The Federal Council of the British Medical Association in Australia, while not sharing all the views expressed by the National Health and Medical Research Council, nevertheless resolved early in 1944 "not to object to the immediate establishment of . . . experimental group practice centres. . . ." [26]

In 1943 the government of New Zealand declared its readiness to build health centers at public expense in regions where physicians would be willing to practice in groups. [27]

The Canadian National Health Act, drafted in 1943, recognized group practice by stating: "Arrangements with medical practitioners . . . may include arrangements with approved clinics, or groups of medical practitioners practising in co-operation, whereby qualified persons may select any such clinic or group of practitioners in lieu of selecting a medical practitioner. . . ." [28]

Group practice is a method with potentialities and limitations. It lends itself to full development in cities and densely populated areas. It can be organized only in a rudimentary way in rural areas with scattered population and poor transportation.

In large communities and densely populated areas, the group should ordinarily include certain specialists as well as general practitioners. The staff as a whole should be responsible for complete service at the home and medical center and, when feasible, also at the general hospital and custodial institution. In many rural areas such organization is difficult, if not impossible, to attain, and general practitioners may be expected to make up the entire group. To bring necessary consultant service to rural groups, arrangements should be made for both organized use, when required, of specialists in the nearest city and regular visits to each group by small teams of consultants.

Location, housing, and equipment of the medical centers should be carefully planned. In general, the centers should be organized on a district basis, with utilization of adequate hospital facilities where this is possible and practicable. In larger communities some of the centers probably could be housed in hospitals or built on their grounds. In smaller communities they would have to be established as independent units and, in many instances, be complemented by infirmaries. To direct the development in proper channels, standards for the building, equipment, and operation of medical centers should be worked out for communities of various sizes.

Group practice often is opposed on the grounds that it precludes free choice of physician.

Ever since there has been organized care of the sick, the medical profession has been fighting for the right of the patient, no matter what his social position, to choose his own doctor; the right of the individual physician to participate in programs for the sick; and the right of the professional association to be consulted in selecting the physicians to be admitted to service. The medical profession has been, and is, maintaining that the preservation of the principle of free choice is basic. Freedom of choice, it is asserted, benefits the patient because confidence in the ability, integrity, and discretion of the physician plays a most important part in the care of the sick; serves the interests of the profession because it offers all competent members opportunity to work; and is to the advantage of the public at large because it safeguards the quality of care. However, even the staunchest supporters of the free choice principle admit limitations upon its application to be indispensable to the successful operation of any program of medical care no matter how it is financed. It is widely acknowledged that the family doctor should be chosen from among those practicing within the geographical area in which the patient resides, that specialists ordinarily should be consulted only on referral from a general practitioner, and that a change from one doctor to another during the same illness or within a certain period of time should be contingent upon presentation of valid reasons.

All these principles can be maintained—and strengthened—by proper organization of group practice.

Obviously if all local physicians work together in a center, the patient is as free to select his family doctor as under the system of individual practice. All he has to do is to state his preference at the center, if he has not already established a relationship before.

If in the same community some physicians belong to groups and others are engaged in individual practice, then, indeed, difficulties may arise. Presuming that free choice is as fundamental as the vast literature and legislative action in its favor indicate, then there cannot be any "ifs" and "buts." A patient who wants to choose a group of physicians as such rather than a doctor in individual practice must be free to do so. Physicians who wish to offer their services as a group must have as much right to participate in a community program as their colleagues conducting their practice in the traditional form. A community must be permitted to select the method of organization best suited to its conditions. Objective interpretation of the principle of free choice precludes its use as an argument against group practice. But it cannot be denied that the operation of group clinics in communities where there are also a number of physicians in individual practice may pose a problem. At its core is the question of competition rather than that of free choice, and this fact must be recognized. The natural way out of this dilemma is to offer the opportunity to practice in groups to all qualified physicians in a community.

To finance the building and equipment of medical centers and to organize the payment for professional services a variety of methods may be employed. There is no innate relationship between group practice and methods of finance. As W. J. Mayo said: "properly considered, group medicine is not a financial arrangement, except for minor details, but a scientific cooperation for the welfare of the sick." [29] However, group practice will only gain in value if the savings it affords are passed on to the "consumer."

PLANNING FOR PAYMENT FOR FACILITIES AND SERVICES

Financing of the construction, equipment, and improvement of medical care facilities and payment for the use of institutional and professional services may be organized in various ways. Two basic methods of organizing payment, both already employed to varying extents, are being weighed at present wherever plans are made to realize the ideal of equal opportunity for good medical care. One is the application of the principle of taxation, the other the application of the principle of insurance. Is there such a thing as "the best method"? To answer this fundamental question the characteristics, potentialities, limitations, and implications of each method must be considered.

Taxation

Public funds for the support of medical care may be obtained by general taxation, special taxation, or both in combination. At present the first system is used widely and the second occasionally. Particularly important in connection with planning for medical care is the fact that various types of taxes affect persons in different economic groups to a quite different extent.

Where revenues are raised through taxes on property and income, which is the prevailing policy at present, individuals and corporations with substantial property, high income, or both pay larger sums and—under the progressive system of taxation—a greater share of their resources than people with little property and small incomes. A substantial fraction of the population has no business with the tax collector. Where excise taxes—such as sales, liquor, beverage, and tobacco taxes—are levied, every consumer contributes to the financing of common tasks, and the more so the more he purchases. Inevitably, the people in the lowest income groups are hit hardest. Ironically, the revenues from liquor and tobacco taxes, in some areas used for support of public medical care, are substantial when consumption is heavy—with the resultant effect of increased incapacitating mental and physical disorders.

Whatever the method of raising revenues, taxation as such is distinguished by certain attributes. Ordinarily, the payments made by individuals in various socio-economic groups are in inverse proportion to their need for medical care. They are not linked to the service the payer may expect. In the mind of the beneficiary, they are not identified with the medical care actually received. Consequently, personal interest in and sense of responsibility for the tax-supported program may be lacking. Groups may be inclined to fight for privileges and rights without thinking of the corresponding duty to the community. They may come to live in a delusion "that the public purse is bottomless," to paraphrase a recent statement by the Canadian Minister of Pensions and National Health.[30]

In using tax revenues for the support of medical care various policies may be pursued. Under the broadest application of the principle of taxation, all facilities and services necessary for adequate medical care would be established and maintained out of public funds.

They would be available without charge to everybody, to the big taxpayer as well as the indigent. Those who carry the burden of costs would also be direct beneficiaries of the service if they so desired.

Under limited application of the principle of taxation, certain types of facilities or services may be singled out for establishment and maintenance at public expense, or selected services may be provided free for designated socio-economic groups. In the first case, each taxpayer shares in the support of public facilities such as hospitals and clinics, whether he uses them or not. Indirectly, if not also directly, he is benefited by the availability of community facilities. In the second case, those who pay taxes finance services to selected groups who usually include self-supporting people as well as persons dependent upon public aid. They discharge their duty to their fellow citizens, without, in most instances, expecting to receive care themselves.

Following this policy public agencies in the United States in 1941 spent approximately 600 to 700 million dollars of tax revenues on the support of medical facilities and services for the civilian population.

A program of public medical care for all, frequently referred to as "all-out state medicine," implies that every resident is eligible for service because he is a resident. If conducted throughout the country, it requires special decisions on admission to the service only when non-residents are in need of aid.

Operation of limited programs, on the other hand, makes it inevitable to define the conditions under which medical care at public expense shall be made available. Qualification for free service may be acquired automatically by employment with a public agency or by service with the armed forces, to mention the most frequent conditions only. It may be granted to individuals "in need" and, then, necessarily involves a "means test." Even if eligibility is determined with sympathy and understanding the approach as such is open to serious objections. It is based on application for aid—the very thing the self-respecting citizen tries to avoid if he can help it. It implies that the applicant and his family have to exhaust most, if not all, of their own resources before they can be accepted for a service that, in the final analysis, is a "last resort." Whether the milk of human kindness flows in a broad gentle stream or merely trickles, charity—well intended as it is—is not what the common man wants. Repayment for the services received, a frequent requirement, may for years severely burden the individual struggling to regain his economic independence after his illness. The patient who needs and demands medical care but is declared ineligible for service at public expense finds neither help nor consolation in the knowledge that his resources, small as they may be, still exceed the limit set by the administration. Thus, restriction of public medical care to persons in need jeopardizes preventive action. It comes too late to prevent complications, serious illness, and chronic stages of sickness. It comes too late to make the most economical use of taxpayers' money. Moreover, the theory of service for persons in need lends itself to policies that are inimical to community planning. As new needs arise, or old ones are realized, new programs are certain to be set up, each designed and operated for one socio-economic group, with a multitude of separate services and agencies the ultimate result. By their very nature limited schemes are exposed to the vagaries of political opinion and pressure. The services may be curtailed by a legislature anxious to please the taxpayer. They may be boosted beyond reasonable limits if votes and political power are at stake. As the funds must be allocated every year, an atmosphere of unrest and instability is created, and this exerts a deleterious influence on the operation of the medical care program.

The principle of tax support for medical care does not necessarily imply a radical change in the nature of medicine and medical care facilities, nor does it embody a sweeping political formula. Tax revenues may be used to pay for public services exclusively, or for nongovernmental as well as governmental health activities. The bearing of this method of finance on the private health professions and voluntary facilities depends on the extent to which it is employed.

Under a system of "all-out state medicine" most, or all, of the members of the health professions would become civil servants. Private practice, if allowed to continue, would have to rely on the demand and purchasing power of a relatively small fraction of the population. Many, or all, of the medical care facilities would become public property. Those owned by nongovernmental organizations, if legally permitted to operate, would be faced with constant financial difficulties and gradually disappear.

If the "middle-road" policy is followed in expending tax funds for medical care, the practice of medicine in form and substance remains a private profession. Nongovernmental institutions and organizations are preserved. Moreover, the private practitioners and the voluntary institutions are sustained, because they receive payment from public agencies for capital expenditures, services furnished to designated groups, or both. To many, the allocations of public funds for expansion or improvement of physical plants or purchase of modern equipment may mean the one chance to keep pace with progress. To many, regular payment for service rendered may well become an important source of income.

From the community point of view employment of public funds for selected activities may be of far-reaching importance. It offers a unique opportunity to coordinate governmental and nongovernmental facilities and services and, thus, paves the way for effective planning of health service.

According to established rules of sound administration, public funds must be administered by public agencies. Consequently, the use of tax revenues to support medical care implies public administration of the sums expended, no matter who is the recipient.

In theory, the method of taxation is conducive to the development of an administrative organization which places responsibility for all tax-supported health services in a single public agency, locally and centrally, and, in addition, links governmental and nongovernmental health activities. In practice, the good chance of setting up such administration usually is missed, but this is not the fault of the method of taxation.

Insurance

Insurance against the economic hazards of sickness, injury, and maternity is a method of pooling risks and resources in order to budget and pay the costs of medical care and/or compensate for loss of earnings due to disability.

The principle of insurance implies that many people must band together under a single plan in order to spread their risks; and they must make small regular prepayments into a common fund in order to pool their resources. The prepayments ordinarily are made out of current income and, when feasible, collected through pay-roll deduction. Although they may be graded according to the earnings of the contributors, they "are or should be related to the value of the benefits and not to capacity to pay," as Sir William Beveridge has stated.[31] The contributions represent savings for a special purpose.

Thus "health insurance" is organized self-help to remove, or reduce, the financial burden which may arise from sickness, injury, or maternity. People can budget and pay for services and cash benefits when they are well and earning. They can obtain service to prevent illness and incapacity for work and receive medical care and compensation for disability when they are sick and disabled.

Contributions may be raised on a voluntary basis or may be legally required of certain groups of the population. In either case, the total amount of the regular prepayments may be divided between employees and employers. Such extension of the cost-sharing principle renders it possible to tap, assemble, and put to effective use the resources of a large number of individuals and families who are accustomed to make some expenditures for medical care but are unable to pay the full cost.

Funds obtained through the device of insurance may be used to provide protection against a variety of hazards, some directly and others indirectly related to health. The first group comprises sickness; accident; maternity; temporary disability due to sickness, accident, and maternity; permanent disability due to sickness and accident; and death due to sickness and accident. In the second group fall old age and unemployment. All or a varying combination of these hazards may be covered by one or several correlated schemes.

Insurance programs may be established for selected economic or occupational groups and thus include a minority of the population. They may be organized for all those able to contribute and thus exclude a minority. In return for contributions the individuals may receive services, cash benefits, or both.

A service plan may be limited in scope, providing for one or a few of the basic types of service—at worst only for "a bottle of medicine and a general practitioner"—or may be inclusive, furnishing all types of service needed. It may be limited in the amount of care, period, or both, or may be operated without any such restrictions.

Cash benefits may be paid to cover specified expenses such as medical or hospital bills; to compensate the insured for loss of income due to sickness, accident, or maternity; or for the two purposes together. The amount of benefit may or may not be fixed in proportion to the size of the contributions. As a general rule it does not exceed a certain limit per type of care, case of illness, or both. The period of payment usually is restricted.

Properly organized insurance plans, and in particular social insurance schemes, have inherent qualities that merit special attention. The group resources are for direct and exclusive use of the members of the group. Contributor and beneficiary are identical. Clearly defined services and cash benefits are made available as of right on the basis of membership, without investigation into the economic conditions of the family and without recovery of costs. Equal advantages are offered to all who are eligible, regardless of their social and economic status. Because of easy access to early diagnosis and early and thorough treatment the frequency of serious stages of illness, complications, and chronic conditions is reduced, the fear of want is removed, and, to a large extent, want is prevented. As the individuals "are kept in touch by their contributions with the actual cost of the service they receive," [32] they are constantly reminded of their own responsibility for efficient and economical operation of the program.

As early as 1825, the advantages obtainable to the individual by insurance have been clearly recognized and admirably stated by a committee of the British House of Commons in the following words:

Whenever there is a contingency, the cheapest way of providing against it is by uniting with others, so that each man may subject himself to a small deprivation, in order that no man may be subjected to a great loss. He, upon whom the contingency does not fall, does not get his money back again, nor does he get for it any visible or tangible benefit; but he obtains security against ruin and consequent peace of mind. He, upon whom the contingency does fall, gets all that those, whom fortune has exempted from it, have lost in hard money, and is thus enabled to sustain an event which would otherwise overwhelm him.[33]

Health insurance is a device with limitations as well as potentialities. It is unsuited to cope with such catastrophes as widespread and severe epidemics, and to meet all the needs arising out of serious and prolonged sickness, such as mental illness and tuberculosis. An insurance program is feasible only for people able to make regular contributions. Even under the most favorable employment and income conditions, there are certain to be persons who have to depend upon public aid for maintenance and, also, self-supporting individuals and families with many children who cannot make more than a token payment, if any, toward the cost of an adequate program of medical care. In periods of slackening business and low incomes, not to mention severe economic crises, the number and proportion of such people is bound to increase substantially. Finally, administrative difficulties may preclude effective operation of an insurance program in thinly settled areas.

To provide the medical care to which the people covered by health insurance are entitled, the services of physicians, dentists, and related groups as well as of institutional facilities must be systematized.

Professional services may be organized in a variety of ways. Any member of the health professions in private practice may be admitted to the program if he so desires, provided he satisfies certain professional and personal requirements, or a definite number may be appointed to full-time positions. In either case, individual practice or group practice may be chosen, depending upon the conditions prevailing in a certain area.

Hospital care may be furnished by selected facilities or by any hospital willing to participate in the service and meeting standards of adequacy, whether it be public or nongovernmental.

This outline, broadly summarizing policies actually followed in a score of countries, shows that health insurance, contrary to assertions frequently made, is not incompatible with private practice nor prejudicial to voluntary hospitals. Actually, it serves the economic interests of both the health professions and the medical care facilities. Payments from insurance organizations are certain and predictable. There are no losses in collection due to "bad debts." Receipts from insurance organizations may become a major source of income for physicians, dentists, pharmacists, and other groups as well as for general and certain special hospitals when a large proportion of the population is covered by the program. Furthermore, with health insurance physicians and dentists can settle in areas otherwise unable to support them.

As a general rule, voluntary health insurance programs are administered by nongovernmental organizations but supervised by public authorities. Responsibility for administration of compulsory schemes may be vested in special statutory bodies—public corporations without the powers of a government authority—or in public agencies. The first method has been given preference in the past. It is considered for introduction by the Canadian government and suggested by the Federal Council of the British Medical Association in Australia.

If administration of compulsory health insurance is separated from that of tax-supported health services, a "state within the state" is created, with friction and waste of administrative effort the inevitable result. The disadvantages of divided authority can be—and often are—lessened but not eliminated by the establishment of associations composed of representatives of the health insurance administration, public agencies, and voluntary organizations engaged in health service. Such associations were increasingly formed in Germany under the Weimar Republic.[34]

Single Method and Combination of Methods

As has been shown in the preceding sections the method of taxation can be of great importance to the systematic building, equipment, and improvement of hospitals and medical centers. There is no substitute for taxation if adequate medical care is to be provided for the millions who have to rely on public aid for their livelihood. However, a system dependent upon a means test for its operation is not an acceptable solution to the problem of financing a sound, constructive program of medical care. The principle of insurance, while free of the shortcomings of taxation, is limited in applicability.

It appears, then, that there is only one single method that would avoid the disadvantages inherent in other approaches to the problem of organizing payment for facilities and services: Public medical care for all, with every necessary service provided as a right and free of charge. Such a system exists in Russia.

Time and again physicians as well as laymen have questioned the wisdom of adopting—or continuing—health insurance. They maintain that the way to a satisfactory program of medical care is by the straight path of all-inclusive state medicine and not by the winding road of health insurance.

Those who advocate a general system of public medical care, or state medicine, offer an array of arguments in favor of their idea. The health professions should not be expected to make a livelihood out of human misery and to compete financially for patients. They should not act as tax collectors, charging the well-to-do "what the traffic can bear" so they can give low-cost or free service to people with small or no means. A system of state medicine would make it possible to provide complete and good medical care for everybody according to his need, rather than his ability to pay. It would be easy to set up, administer, and supervise, and it would be economical in operation. Personnel and facilities could be distributed according to the requirements of various sections of the country. The health professions would gain economic security and an opportunity to keep abreast of scientific progress through regular leaves of absence for postgraduate study and research. The latest example of a proposal based on this reasoning is the plan advocated by the Australian National Health and Medical Research Council.[35]

The opponents of a general system of public medical care stress two major facts that militate against its adoption. Much of the burden of financing the service would be placed on those who have considerable income and property. New and heavy levies on a minority of the population might well defeat their own purpose by forcing liquidation of assets to pay taxes. Furthermore, the introduction of public medical care would necessarily carry with it the establishment of a full-time salaried medical service and sound the death knell of private practice. Such policy would "not be in the best interests of the community," to quote frequent statements. "Once get medicine under the control of the Civil Service and 'good-bye' to the best that medicine can do. It may be all right for a good many other callings, but to medicine it will be fatal to efficiency," Lord Dawson of Penn recently declared in a discussion of British plans. Quantity and cost of service would receive primary attention and the quality of medical care would be lowered. As Scottish authors said, the system "might at one point militate strongly against the full application of modern conceptions of medicine."[36] Promotions and transfers would involve frequent changes of personnel, with the result that the physicians would not acquire intimate knowledge of the families. There would be no personal relationship between patient and physician, nor freedom to choose and change the doctor. Bureaucratic control would spell regimentation of physicians. It would kill the spirit of adventure, initiative, and freedom to act. Political influences would play a detrimental role in selecting personnel, furnishing service, and administering the program.

While strong opposition against full-time salaried medical service has been registered by the majority of the medical professions in many countries, the disapproval is not unqualified. That such a system is necessary in sparsely settled areas, poor districts, and small communities with rural hinterland is not denied. To give a few examples, full-time salaried medical service is steadily expanding in parts of Australia, primarily in the Northern Territory, Queensland, and Tasmania,[37] and well-established in several Canadian "municipalities." [38]

If a general system of public medical care is rejected, combination of taxation and insurance logically moves into the center of deliberations. Basically, the two methods are complementary rather than conflicting. If they are properly applied, each for the achievement of clearly defined ends, an effective instrument for service to the community can be produced.

For what purposes and how far should the method of taxation be employed?

Taxation should be used primarily for the building and development of adequate medical care facilities, whenever there is proven need for them and other resources are lacking. If a well-organized program of medical care is established or planned, no valid reason exists for public agencies to be reluctant in spending tax funds also on nongovernmental buildings serving community purposes. Insurance funds ordinarily should not be utilized for capital expenditures. Special conditions, such as those prevailing in large industrial plants, may justify exceptions to this rule. Such policy follows from the assumption that medical care facilities should be established and operated for all rather than the selected groups who contribute to the insurance scheme.

As a method of paying for service to civilians taxation should play a subsidiary role. In general, public funds should be allotted for three specific purposes: to provide medical care for persons depending upon public aid for maintenance; to furnish service to war veterans with service-connected diseases or disabilities; and to lower hospital rates for patients with communicable diseases.

Extension of public medical care to self-supporting persons is a stopgap, explained but not excused by the lack of organized self-help. The policy of "gradualism," of inching along and patching up as emergencies arise, perpetuates and intensifies the old evils of categorical approach, inequality of service, and diffusion of authority. What is needed is not expansion but reduction of the system of relief to the utmost possible minimum. What is necessary is not reform where there is no reasonable chance for it but recovery from the idea that society has obligations for the needy only.

Compulsory health insurance is the only method capable of "relieving" the relief system because it alone is applicable to marginal income groups as well as others. With such a scheme public medical care can be confined to a relatively small fraction of the population whose need for public aid will persist because there is no employable member in the family. As has been shown time and again social insurance in general and health insurance in particular markedly affect "poor relief" and public assistance for special groups. They decrease the number of persons who have to turn to public agencies for support, although they cannot end public assistance. The larger the part of the population covered, the more complete the medical care and the higher the cash benefits provided by a national social insurance scheme—the smaller the number of applications for assistance at public expense. The more limited the coverage, medical care, and cash benefits of social insurance the heavier need and demand for public medical care among that large number of self-supporting families and individuals who cannot afford good medical care at private rates.

Without social insurance including health insurance the extension of public medical care is inevitable, despite the admitted shortcomings of such a policy. Even if truly adequate programs of voluntary health insurance were to exist throughout the country, the contributions necessary to make them self-sustaining would be too high for a large proportion of the population.

Some thirty countries have come to adopt the combination of compulsory insurance and taxation for the organized payment of medical care. Some more, including the United States and Canada, are studying legislative measures to this effect.

Bills under consideration in various countries are identical in recommending the use of social insurance and taxation in conjunction. They differ in their proposals on the application of the principle of taxation.

The British plan for a National Health Service, designed primarily to improve the existing program of compulsory health insurance, includes allocation of tax funds for the support of voluntary as well as public hospitals and for the medical care of persons receiving public assistance.[39]

The Wagner-Murray-Dingell Bill ("The Social Security Act Amendments of 1943"), introduced in the United States Congress, would establish health insurance, including "medical and hospitalization insurance benefits," maternity insurance, and temporary and permanent disability insurance; extend the coverage of the present scheme of old-age insurance; and unify unemployment insurance. In addition it would provide for the allotment of tax funds to the states to support medical care for recipients of general assistance, a policy already followed for the benefit of persons accepted for old-age assistance, aid to dependent children, and aid to the blind. But the legislative draft does not contain any provision for the building, equipment, and improvement of hospitals and medical centers out of public funds.[40]

The Wagner-Murray-Dingell Bill, like the Canadian bill, would enable public agencies to make payments on behalf of the needy to the administration of social insurance.

Despite the employment of different payment methods medical care should be the same for all. To achieve this, health service should be divorced from public assistance as such. While public assistance authorities should pay for the care of the needy by making regular contributions to the social insurance scheme, they should discontinue operation and administration of services of their own. Such a policy would not only offer vast opportunities to equalize and standardize medical care but attain much more. It would eliminate the need for transfer of patients from one system to another and thereby assure continuity of care. It would remove any justification for the maintenance of separate administrations of medical care programs for numerous groups and thus simplify the administrative machinery. It would be an added inducement to abolish residence and settlement requirements. The only risk involved in such a procedure is the shock to those who cling to the tradition of the poor law.

Cash Payment to the Sick for Medical Care Expenses

Whether it be taxation or insurance that furnish the funds for the payment of medical care, the individual should be provided with service rather than money. Cash payment defeats its own purpose, as

PLANNING FOR MEDICAL CARE

abundant experience has shown. Four arguments against this method deserve special mention.

1. Attainment of early diagnosis and complete treatment is impeded. To control the expenditures, the total amount allowable in the individual case as well as the reimbursement for specified types of care must be restricted.

2. Quality of medical care is hard to improve, as merely a kind of bank arrangement is made.

3. Unnecessary service is encouraged. The sick may want to take advantage of their privilege up to the limit even if there is no medical indication. The health professions and medical care facilities may be tempted to extend their services in an effort to please their patients.

4. The money paid out to the beneficiaries may be spent unwisely, for instance on drugs not prescribed, or even for purposes for which it is not intended.

Realizing the shortcomings of the method of cash payment, Congress, in appropriating money for Emergency Maternity and Infant Care, stated that the funds were to provide medical care. As the United States Children's Bureau explained in a memorandum to the states: "The payment of direct grants to the wives of enlisted men could give no assurance that the funds would be used to provide . . . care as specified by Congress. Appropriations . . . can be expended only by the State health agencies actually to purchase . . . care." [41]

The Wagner-Murray-Dingell Bill would make it legally permissible for the Federal government to allot funds to states furnishing assistance to needy individuals in the form of medical care. Thus, the former restrictions, so widely criticized, would be abolished.[42]

PLANNING FOR ADMINISTRATION OF MEDICAL CARE

Good administrative organization of medical care requires (1) clear definition of the powers and functions of the responsible agencies; (2) professional direction and supervision of professional matters; (3) organized participation of the health professions, the representatives of medical care facilities, and of the "consumers" of medical service; and (4) coordination of the health service administration with governmental agencies responsible for fields of activity indirectly related to health, and with voluntary health and welfare organizations.

The past carries the plain lesson that future legislation dealing with medical care must embody these four basic principles and outline the policies and procedures necessary to implement them. Yet, many of the current plans for the improvement of medical care, bold as they are in regard to organization and payment of facilities and services, are anything but adventurous with respect to administrative organization. Their omissions are as eloquent as their suggestions. It is not so much the newness of the science and art of health administration as the fear of the political dynamite in the matter that causes the marked reluctance to touch the subject.

To arrive at a sound decision on the administrative powers and functions of the agencies responsible for medical care, the basic issue of centralization or decentralization must be settled in a way suited to the special requirements of health service. Theoretically three solutions of the problem are possible: (1) centralization of both power and function; (2) decentralization of both power and function; and (3) centralization of power, complete or limited, along with decentralization of function or certain types of function. Each of these possibilities has advantages and disadvantages.

The first approach makes it possible to organize and finance a nation-wide system of medical care with uniform standards for personnel, facilities, services, and administration in every section of the country; and to direct its organic growth, supervise its execution, and enforce pertinent statutes and administrative rules. On the debit side must be listed the grave dangers of regimentation and remote control of local activities—dangers that may become a real threat to the effective operation and sound development of the program.

Complete autonomy at the local level enables localities with sufficient resources to set up and administer their own medical care programs according to local needs and conditions. But the power of self-government may be exercised by localities to quite a different extent, depending not only on their wealth but also on town-hall politics. It may become a paper proposition when taxable income is low. At best adequate service may be provided by a smaller or larger fraction of all localities, with qualitative and quantitative inequality of service and costly administration the inevitable result. At worst serious shortcomings in health service as well as administrative chaos may dominate the national picture.

Centralization of precisely stated powers together with decentralization of clearly defined functions offers an unparalleled opportunity to develop the best features of centralization and also preserve and strengthen self-government where it can be of greatest value. The problem then is to divide and balance the powers of central and local authorities and to distribute their functions in a manner which serves to attain adequate health service.

The difficulty of arriving at a satisfactory solution is great. Proposals formulated from the expert point of view may be defeated on political grounds, as intricate questions of Federal-state, state-county, and county-town relations are involved. A poor compromise may be offered and accepted for the sake of expediency—and a good principle be corrupted.

Past experience supports the conclusion that centralization of certain powers in conjunction with decentralization of certain functions deserves primary attention in planning the framework of the administrative structure. In principle, the central authority should have power to formulate nation-wide policies in regard to organization, payment, and administration of medical care; set standards for personnel, facilities, services, and administrative organization; lend technical assistance to the agencies in charge of direct administration; give financial assistance to the responsible administrative units, the funds to be allotted in inverse relation to the wealth of the areas; coordinate the local activities; and supervise adequacy and economy of service. Except for special conditions the central authority should administer only highly specialized facilities and services infrequently needed by individual communities and general and special hospitals serving several political units. A modification of this principle may be necessary in countries which are a federation of states with constitutional rights of their own. In that case Federal-state cooperation on the basis of nationally established standards would have to be emphasized. The states would be vested with the power and charged with the duty to do within their jurisdiction what the Federal government does for the nation as a whole.

With the exceptions stated before, administration of direct service should be decentralized and delegated to units large enough to assure effective and economical administration. This implies regional organization of the entire medical care administration throughout the country, with incorporation of this principle into the law of the land. "To allow units of historical interest only to override functional need is certain to lead to inefficiency," as the authors of Medical Planning

Research stressed.[43] Regions convenient for proper administrative effort may be created by dividing large political units, such as states or provinces, into medical service areas cutting across state lines as well as county lines, if necessary. In each functional area, in addition to one central office, a sufficient number of branch offices should be set up close to the individuals to be served.

The vertical administrative organization outlined here must be accompanied by an appropriate horizontal organization. Otherwise its value would be greatly impaired. Centrally as well as locally a single agency should be responsible at least for all tax-supported services, whether preventive or curative, and, if feasible, also for medical care under social insurance. To achieve this, existing public agencies or divisions whose purposes run parallel must be consolidated. Judging from the experience of the past this ideal may be impossible to realize. If drastic measures are refused before a malady becomes incurable, symptomatic treatment to mitigate its effects is the logical alternative. Applied to administration of medical care this means that the old iron fences separating the multitude of public agencies concerned with medical care ought to be scrapped and coordination of administration be organized. Coordination, however, may involve establishment of new bodies such as interdepartmental committees. It operates slowly, uncertainly and, often, inadequately, being what it is: a typical "Ersatz" product.

If professional direction and supervision of the technical and professional aspects of medical care is to be developed properly, two general principles must be accepted and generally applied. To assure competence of professional personnel, appointments to administrative positions should be made strictly on the basis of merit and, when feasible, through competitive examinations. This rule should be observed for all: physicians, dentists, pharmacists, medical social workers, public health nurses, and other groups. To enable the appointees to concentrate on their administrative work, the positions should be full-time and protected by the right of tenure. Under regional organization of medical care administration, part-time appointments will be warranted but infrequently. If they cannot be avoided, physicians, dentists, and similar professional persons charged with administrative duties should not be permitted to accept patients covered by the program. The classification of the positions, the salary rates, and the possibilities of grade promotions should be such as to attract capable professional persons willing to make administration of medical care a career.

It would be inconsistent to promote the idea of professional direction and supervision without stressing the urgent need for training of specialists in medical care administration. It might happen that aptness comes with the office. But it is certain that qualification for highly specialized work can best be acquired by special preparation, both theoretical and practical. A selected number of schools of medicine, public health, and social work should include in their plans of instruction courses, seminars, and field work in organization and administration of medical care.[44] Other appropriate institutions should offer courses for persons interested in sub-professional, clerical, and similar positions with administrative agencies.

The British government's document on National Health Service states "there is room for special devices to secure that the guidance of the expert is available and does not go unheeded. Otherwise the quality of the service is bound to suffer." To translate this idea into practice the British plan proposes the establishment of a Central Health Services Council, a "statutory body" designed to be "the mouthpiece of expert opinion."[45] Following the same line of thought the Wagner-Murray-Dingell Bill in the United States contains a provision for the creation of a "National Advisory Medical and Hospital Council."[46] These two examples are typical of a definite trend toward organization of close cooperation between governmental agencies responsible for medical care and the various groups rendering service.

Experience already made with the institution of advisory committees indicates how they should be organized to be most useful.

Advisory committees should be formed centrally and locally. They should be regularly consulted by governmental agencies, but the expert bodies should also be free to express their views on their own initiative. To promote effective cooperation the advisory committees should be composed of representatives of (1) the physicians, dentists, pharmacists, nurses, and medical social workers; (2) the governmental and nongovernmental hospitals, including teaching hospitals; (3) the public agencies responsible for fields related to health service; (4) the voluntary organizations engaged in health and welfare activities, in so far as practical; and (5) the general public, including all important "consumer" groups. Technical subcommittees should be set up for major groups or special assignments.

The functions of the committees should be broadly defined. They should include advice on the organization of professional services and medical care facilities, payment methods, and principles of administration—with particular emphasis on problems of adequacy and economy of service—and be extended to program planning as well as to development and operation of the service.

It is a pious platitude that cooperation of health agencies with others providing service to the individual can contribute much to the efficacy and economy of the total plan. But it is also true that in actual practice this matter receives but insufficient attention.

The agencies administering health service should do everything in their power to establish a working relationship with public agencies and voluntary organizations active in such fields as welfare, education, including vocational training, housing, and employment service. There are few areas of human activities in which the superiority of concerted action over isolated effort is as evident as in health service.

UNDERLYING PHILOSOPHY

Planning for adequate medical care is more than a method of organizing the application of scientific knowledge and technical skill. It is the expression of a social philosophy. It is effective only in so far as it is sustained by a conviction of principle.

The philosophy underlying modern health policy rests on two cornerstones: society's need of the fit and productive individual and the individual's right to health. This concept recognizes the reciprocity of health and economy; the interdependence of the individual and the state as well as their mutual obligations; and the need for social action substituting solidarity for isolated individual effort.

Such ideas have long been inherent in our political philosophy. For generations they have guided the development of certain health activities, particularly sanitation of the environment. But it was only in recent times that they were applied to the whole field of health service.

In 1929, Franklin Delano Roosevelt, said: "Fifty years ago, the matter of health was individual; it was nobody's concern, except that of the family, whether a person was healthy or not, and gradually we have built up a new doctrine—the belief that the State has a positive right, not just an obligation, to see that the health of its individuals is brought up to a higher level. . . . The State is going to insist, fifty years from now, on good health, insist on it as a right of what is known as the sovereignty of the people." [47]

Going a step farther, the Committee of Physicians for the Improvement of Medical Care, in 1937, not only reaffirmed the then widely accepted tenet "the health of the people is a direct concern of the government" but recommended "that a national health policy directed toward all groups of the population should be formulated." [48]

One of the most comprehensive statements ever made by any legislative body came from a subcommittee of the United States Senate reporting on the Wagner Bill of 1939. This measure contained a series of proposals for the improvement of health service, including introduction of compulsory insurance against temporary disability and of a general program of medical care. In its preliminary report the subcommittee declared: "The first interest of an enlightened government is the well-being of its citizens, and health is a fundamental element in well-being. . . . The most important asset of our Nation is the health of our citizens, for upon health and vigor depends their economic capacity to be productive. . . . Just as health is the most precious possession of the individual, so is the healthy citizenry the most precious possession of a nation. Poor health leads to unhappiness, poverty, dependency, and even to crime; good health contributes to well-being, production, income, and wealth. The ideals and principles of American democracy call for equality of opportunity. Such equality of opportunity certainly cannot exist unless all groups in the population have access to those health services needed to prevent and cure disease, and to promote vitality and well-being." [49]

While the "positive right" of the state to safeguard the health of its citizens is a fairly recent concept, the right of the individual to health has its roots in a far earlier period. The Declaration of Independence enunciated the fundamental democratic tenet that men possess the natural rights of life, liberty, and the pursuit of happiness. By tacit consent these words have been interpreted as including the "right to health" and, thus, the right to medical care. The French Constitution of June 24, 1793, declared formally: "Public aid is a sacred duty. Society is obliged to provide subsistence for the underprivileged."

With the evolution of democratic thought its individual doctrines, particularly those of equality, freedom, and social justice, have assumed new meanings. Abstract objectives are being redefined and clarified in the light of the needs and potentialities of our present civilization.

The Atlantic Charter of August 14, 1941, which signalized the great resurgence of the democratic faith under the blows struck by the united forces of brutalitarianism, proclaimed "Freedom from Fear and Want" as one of the common principles on which the United Nations based their "'hopes for a better future for the world."

The modern "Bill of Rights" postulates "the right to adequate food, clothing, shelter and medical care." [50] From H. G. Wells in England to the National Resources Planning Board in the United States we find expressions of the same concept, and in the "Medical Care Recommendation" adopted by the International Labor Conference in 1944, we possess the first proposal for its international realization.[51]

The acceptance of these ideas lays upon society the responsibility for their execution. There must be equal opportunity for all persons to obtain good medical care. Only by keeping this goal constantly before our eyes can we hope to undertake the long and arduous task of translating philosophy into fact, of shaping fact to the pattern of our philosophy, of making pledge and performance match. In the words of Sir Arthur Newsholme:

"Civilized communities have arrived at two conclusions, from which there will be no retreat, though their full realization in experience has nowhere been completely achieved.

In the first place, THE HEALTH OF EVERY INDIVIDUAL IS A SOCIAL CONCERN AND RESPONSIBILITY; and secondly, as following from this, MEDICAL CARE IN ITS WIDEST SENSE FOR EVERY INDIVIDUAL IS AN ESSENTIAL CONDITION OF MAXIMUM EFFICIENCY AND HAPPINESS IN A CIVILIZED COMMUNITY." [52]

REFERENCES

2: THE GROWTH OF PUBLIC HOSPITALS

1. "Hospital Service in the United States," *Journal of the American Medical Association*, CXXI (March 27, 1943), No. 13, 1010, 1012, 1021.
2. J. H. Harley Williams, *A Century of Public Health in Britain, 1832–1929*, London, 1932, p. 102. Quoted with permission of the publishers, A. & C. Black, Ltd.
3. *Principles of Hospital Administration and the Training of Hospital Executives*, Report of the Committee on the Training of Hospital Executives [Rockefeller Foundation], New York, 1922, pp. 13–14.
4. Henry C. Burdett, *Hospitals and Asylums of the World*, London, 1893, III, 59.
5. Joe Smith, *Kern General Hospital: 1867–1940*, Bakersfield, Cal., 1940, p. 41.
6. M. L. Davis, "Hospital for Contagious and Infectious Diseases," in International Congress of Charities, Correction, and Philanthropy, Section III, *Hospitals, Dispensaries and Nursing*, Baltimore and London, 1894, p. 176. Quoted with permission of the publishers, The Johns Hopkins Press.
7. PEP (Political and Economic Planning), *Report on the British Health Services*, London, 1937, p. 257.
8. U.S. Public Health Service, *The Control of Communicable Diseases*, Reprint No. 1697 from the *Public Health Reports*, rev., 1940.
9. American Hospital Association, Thirty-Third Annual Convention, *Transactions*, XXXIII (1931), 324–32.
10. Karl Sudhoff, "Die ersten Massnahmen der Stadt Nürnberg gegen die Syphilis in den Jahren 1496 und 1497," *Archiv für Dermatologie und Syphilis*, CXVI (1913), No. 1, 7.
11. G. H. M. Rowe, "Isolating Wards and Hospitals for Infectious Diseases," in International Congress of Charities, Correction, and Philanthropy, Section III, *Hospitals, Dispensaries and Nursing*, p. 135. Quoted with permission of the publishers, The Johns Hopkins Press.
12. Hermann Brehmer, *Die Gesetze der Entstehung und des Fortschreitens der Lungen-Tuberkulose*, Berlin, 1853.

13. Hermann Brehmer, *Die chronische Lungenschwindsucht und Tuberkulose der Lunge, ihre Ursache und ihre Heilung*, Berlin, 1857; rev. ed., Berlin, 1869.
14. Edward L. Trudeau, *An Autobiography*, Philadelphia and New York, 1916.
15. "Tuberculosis Facilities in the United States," *Journal of the American Medical Association*, CXIV (March 2, 1940), No. 9, 766–69.
16. U.S. Bureau of the Census, "Hospital and Other Institutional Facilities and Services," *Vital Statistics—Special Reports*, XIII (March 2, 1942), No. 53, 539.
17. Interdepartmental Committee to Coordinate Health and Welfare Activities, *The Need for a National Health Program*, Washington, D.C., 1938, p. 32.
18. Philip P. Jacobs, *The Control of Tuberculosis in the United States*, New York, 1932, pp. 111–13.
19. Robert Koch, "Epidemiologie der Tuberkulose," *Zeitschrift für Hygiene und Infektionskrankheiten*, LXVII (1910), No. 1, 17.
20. Franz Goldmann, "Die Dauerunterbringung ansteckend Tuberkulöser," *Archiv für Soziale Hygiene und Demographie*, I (1926), No. 3, 231–38.
21. Sir P. C. Varrier-Jones, "Village Settlements for the Tuberculous," Mitchell Lecture, 1927, Royal College of Physicians, London; and "The Economics of After-Care in Tuberculosis," *British Journal of Tuberculosis*, XXIV (Oct., 1931), No. 4, 175–81.
22. Elliott H. Pennell, Joseph W. Mountin, and Kay Pearson, "Financial Support of Hospitals Controlled by State and Local Governments," *Public Health Reports*, LVI (March 7, 1941), No. 10, 433–45.
23. The Body of Liberties of the Colony of Massachusetts Bay, 1641.
24. Albert Deutsch, *The Mentally Ill in America: A History of Their Care and Treatment from Colonial Times*, New York, 1937.
25. Henry Harris, *California's Medical Story*, Springfield, Ill., 1932, p. 116.
26. Isabel C. Bruce and Edith Eickhoff, *The Michigan Poor Law*, University of Chicago Social Service Monographs, No. 23, Chicago, 1936, p. 76. Quoted with permission of the publishers, The University of Chicago Press.
27. MS Minutes, New York Hospital, as quoted by John Brett Langstaff, *Doctor Bard of Hyde Park*, New York, 1942, p. 113. Quoted with permission of the publishers, E. P. Dutton & Co., Inc.

28. U.S. Bureau of the Census, "Psychiatric Services in General Hospitals: 1941," *Vital Statistics—Special Reports*, XV (June 5, 1942), No. 28, 337-38.
29. Dorothea Lynde Dix, *Memorial to the Legislature of Massachusetts*, Boston, 1843, p. 4.
30. Clifford W. Beers, *A Mind That Found Itself: An Autobiography*, New York and London, 1908.
31. U.S. Bureau of the Census. "Patients in Hospitals for Mental Disease: 1939," *Vital Statistics—Special Reports*, XV (Jan. 31, 1942), No. 10, 105-20; "Mental Patients in Institutions," *Vital Statistics—Special Reports*, XV (Jan. 20, 1942), No. 9, 89-101.
32. Grover A. Kempf, *Laws Pertaining to the Admission of Patients to Mental Hospitals Throughout the United States*, Supplement No. 157 to the *Public Health Reports*, 1939.
    Samuel W. Hamilton, Grover A. Kempf, Grace C. Scholz, and Eve G. Caswell, *A Study of the Public Mental Hospitals of the United States, 1937-1939*, Supplement No. 164 to the *Public Health Reports*, 1941.
33. Joseph W. Mountin and Evelyn Flook, "Distribution of Health Services in the Structure of State Government," Chap. VI, "Medical and Dental Care by State Agencies," *Public Health Reports*, LVII (Aug. 14, 1942), No. 33, 1195-1209.
34. "Hospital Service in the United States," *Journal of the American Medical Association*, CXXI (March 27, 1943), No. 13, 1011, 1015-16.
35. U.S. Bureau of the Census, "Hospital and Other Institutional Facilities and Services," *Vital Statistics—Special Reports*, XIII (March 2, 1942), No. 53, 536-39, 553-54, 577-83.
36. Interdepartmental Committee to Coordinate Health and Welfare Activities, *The Need for a National Health Program*, p. 32.
37. John Brett Langstaff, *Doctor Bard of Hyde Park*, pp. 103-4. Quoted with permission of the publishers, E. P. Dutton & Co., Inc.
38. U.S. Congress, Public Law 137, First Session, Seventy-seventh Congress, June 28, 1941, Title II, Sec. 201.
39. Louis F. Frank, *The Medical History of Milwaukee, 1834-1914*, Milwaukee, 1915, pp. 146, 155.
40. *Annual Report of the Administrator of Veterans' Affairs for the Fiscal Year 1942*, Washington, D.C., pp. 9-10; *Annual Report of the Surgeon General of the Public Health Service of the United States for the Fiscal Year 1942*, Washington, D.C., p. 11.
41. Calculated on the basis of figures given by the American College of Surgeons, *Bulletin*, XXVII (Oct., 1942), No. 4, 245-335.

42. Michael M. Davis and Margaret L. Plumley, "Governmental Hospitals—Importance in General Care," *The Modern Hospital*, LIII (July, 1939), No. 1, 76–78.
43. American Hospital Association, Forty-First Annual Convention, *Transactions* XLI (1939), 476.
44. *Louisiana Acts 1926*, Act No. 62, Sec. 1.
45. *California Appellate Decisions, 1935–36*, 84, 354.
46. Margaret L. Plumley, "Organization and Financial Policy of City and County Hospitals," American Hospital Association, Forty-First Annual Convention, *Transactions*, XLI (1939), 472–73.
47. Elliott H. Pennell, Joseph W. Mountin, and Kay Pearson, "Financial Support of Hospitals Controlled by State and Local Governments," *Public Health Reports*, LVI (March 7, 1941), No. 10, 436–45.
48. Joseph W. Mountin, Elliott H. Pennell, and Kay Pearson, "Hospitals Existing Singly in Counties Have Similar Financial Structure," *Public Health Reports*, LVI (March 14, 1941), No. 11, 501–8.
49. Michael M. Davis and Margaret L. Plumley, "Small Community Trends," *The Modern Hospital*, LIII (Aug., 1939), No. 2, 57.

3: FROM "FREE DISPENSARY" TO PUBLIC MEDICAL CENTER

1. Margaret L. Plumley, "Location and Characteristics of 769 Out-Patient Departments," *Hospitals*, XI (Dec., 1937), No. 12, 79–85.
2. American Hospital Association, "Ideals and Policies for the Administration of Clinics, Dispensaries or Out-Patient Departments Doing Out-Patient Work," *Transactions*, XXVII (1925), 78–82.
3. American College of Surgeons, *Manual of Hospital Standardization*, Chicago, 1938, pp. 53–55.
4. *A Survey of the Facilities for the Care of the Sick of Rochester, New York*, mimeographed, Rochester, 1941, p. 48.
5. Michael M. Davis, "Out-Patient Service in the United States," in Haven Emerson, ed., *Administrative Medicine*, New York, 1941, pp. 121–33.
6. American Hospital Association, "Ideals and Policies for the Administration of Clinics, Dispensaries or Out-Patient Departments Doing Out-Patient Work," *Transactions*, XXVII (1925), 80.
7. *Ibid.*
8. Emil Frankel "Statistical Analysis of 6600 Out-Patients," *Hospitals*, XV (Sept., 1941), No. 9, 97.

9. Margaret L. Plumley, "Out-Patient Operating Costs," *The Modern Hospital*, XLIX (Dec., 1937), No. 6, 65–67.
10. Margaret L. Plumley, "Location and Characteristics of 769 Out-Patient Departments," *Hospitals*, XI (Dec., 1937), No. 12, 80.
11. Margaret L. Plumley, "Out-Patient Operating Costs," *The Modern Hospital*, XLIX (Dec., 1937), No. 6, 65–66.
12. Henry E. Sigerist, "Medical Care through Medical Centers in the Soviet Union," *American Review of Soviet Medicine*, I (Dec., 1943), No. 2, 176–90.
13. Anthony J. Borowski and Margaret L. Plumley, "Preventive Clinic Facilities Available in 94 Selected Counties of the United States," *Public Health Reports*, LIV (March 3, 1939), No. 5, 335–42.
14. PEP (Political and Economic Planning), *Report on the British Health Services*, London, 1937, pp. 359–62.
15. C.-E. A. Winslow, "A Half-Century of the Massachusetts Public Health Association," *American Journal of Public Health*, XXX (April, 1940), No. 4, 333.
16. Charles F. Wilinsky, "The Health Center," *American Journal of Public Health*, XVII (July, 1927), No. 7, 677–82; and "Dovetailing Health Work," *The Modern Hospital*, XLVII (Sept., 1936), No. 3, 61–63.
17. Haven Emerson, "City Health Center," *The Modern Hospital*, XLIX (Aug., 1937), No. 2, 40.
18. *Ibid.*, 41.
19. Charles F. Wilinsky, "The Health Center," *American Journal of Public Health*, XVII (July, 1927), No. 7, 677.
20. Henry F. Vaughan and Ledru O. Geib, "The Doctor's Office as a Health Center," excerpt in *Tuberculosis Abstracts*, VII (April, 1934), No. 4, 1.
21. National Tuberculosis Association, *Tuberculosis Clinic Manual*, New York, 1938, p. 14.
22. Marion Nelson, "Practice in Tuberculosis Clinics in the United States," *The American Review of Tuberculosis*, XXXVI (Nov., 1937), No. 5, 623.
23. U.S. Public Health Service, *The Principles of Venereal Disease Control*, Supplement No. 17 to *Venereal Disease Information*, Washington, D.C., 1942, p. 20.
24. Franz Goldmann, "Medical Care," *Social Work Year Book 1943*, New York, 1943, p. 308. Quoted with permission of the publishers, Russell Sage Foundation.

25. Committee on Research in Medical Economics, *Group Medical Practice*, New York, 1940, p. 6.
26. Douglas Hubble, "Future of the Family Doctor," *The Lancet*, CCXLIX (Oct. 12, 1940), 461.
27. Grace W. Myers, *History of the Massachusetts General Hospital, June, 1872 to December, 1900*, Boston, 1929, p. 64. Quoted with permission of the publishers, Massachusetts General Hospital.
28. "Report of the Bureau of Medical Economics," *Journal of the American Medical Association*, CXVI (April 19, 1941), No. 16, 1803.
29. American Medical Association, *Principles of Medical Ethics*, Chap. III, Art. VI, Sec. 2.
30. American Medical Association v. United States, 317 U.S. 519 (1943).

4: THE DEVELOPMENT OF PROGRAMS OF PUBLIC MEDICAL CARE FOR "PERSONS IN NEED"

1. J. H. Harley Williams, *A Century of Public Health in Britain, 1832–1929*. London, 1932, p. 4. Quoted with permission of the publishers, A. & C. Black, Ltd.
2. *Ibid.*, p. 20. Quoted with permission of the publishers.
3. Juan-Luis Vivès, *Concerning the Relief of the Poor; or Concerning Human Need*. Translated by Margaret M. Sherwood. The New York School of Philanthropy, Studies in Social Work, No. 11, 1917, p. 6. Quoted with permission of the publishers, The New York School of Social Work, Columbia University.
4. Franz Goldmann, *Recent Developments in Tax-Supported Medical Care in Great Britain*, American Public Welfare Association, Chicago, 1939.
5. Edith Abbott, *Public Assistance*, Chicago, 1940.
6. *Social Security Yearbook, 1941*, p. 30.
7. *Ibid.*
8. William Graham Sumner, "The Forgotten Man," in A. G. Keller, ed., *The Forgotten Man and Other Essays*, New Haven, 1918, p. 476.
9. Committee on the Costs of Medical Care, Twenty-eight Publications. Final Report, *Medical Care for the American People*, Chicago, 1932.
U.S. Public Health Service, *National Health Survey*, Sickness and Medical Care Series, rev. ed., Washington, D.C., 1939.
Social Security Board, *Medical Care and Costs in Relation to*

Family Income, Bureau Memorandum No. 51, Washington, D.C., 1943.

10. Committee of Physicians for the Improvement of Medical Care, *Principles and Proposals*, New Haven, 1937, p. 2.
11. "Proceedings of the Special Session of the House of Delegates," *Journal of the American Medical Association*, CXI (Sept. 24, 1938), No. 13, 1216.
12. "Platform," *Journal of the American Medical Association*, CXIII (Nov. 25, 1939), No. 22, 1966.
13. State of New York, *Session Laws of 1941*, Chap. 82, Sec. 1.
14. State of Rhode Island, *Public Laws of 1942*, Chap. 1212, Art. 1.
15. *Acts and Resolves of Massachusetts, 1937*, Chap. 332, Sec. 67D, as amended May 25, 1939.
16. U.S. Congress, Public Law 11, First Session, Seventy-eighth Congress, March 18, 1943.
17. American Association of Medical Social Workers, *Criteria for Determining Eligibility for Public Medical Care*, Chicago, 1940.
18. "Proceedings of the Special Session of the House of Delegates," *Journal of the American Medical Association*, CXI (Sept. 24, 1938), No. 13, 1215.
19. American Hospital Association, Forty-Fourth Annual Convention, *Transactions*, XLIV (1942), 134.
20. American Public Welfare Association, *Organization and Administration of Tax-Supported Medical Care*, Chicago, 1939, p. 7.
21. U.S. Congress, Public Law 540, Third Session, Seventy-fifth Congress, May 24, 1938.
22. American Public Welfare Association, *Report of the Committee on Medical Care*, Annual Meeting, Seattle, Wash., 1938, p. 26.
23. American Public Welfare Association, *Organization and Administration of Tax-Supported Medical Care*, p. 4.
24. Robert S. Drews, "A History of the Care of the Sick Poor of the City of Detroit (1703–1855)," *Bulletin of the History of Medicine*, VII (July, 1939), No. 7, 764.
25. State of Connecticut, *Report of the Commission to Study the Pauper Laws*, Hartford, 1937, p. 42.
26. Isabel C. Bruce and Edith Eickhoff, *The Michigan Poor Law*, University of Chicago Social Service Monographs, No. 23, Chicago, 1936, pp. 72–87.
27. Robert C. Lowe, *State Public Welfare Legislation*, Works Progress Administration, Division of Research, Research Monograph XX, Washington, D.C., 1939, p. 8.

28. State of Washington, *Session Laws of 1941*, Chap. 1, Par. 15.
29. Edith M. Baker, "Crippled Children," *Social Work Year Book 1941*, New York, 1941, pp. 162–63.
30. State of Tennessee, *Public Acts 1939*, Chap. 102, Sec. 4.
31. New York State Department of Social Welfare, *Analytical Chart of Reimbursable Medical, Dental and Nursing Care*, Sept. 28, 1942, p. 1.
32. Chicago Relief Administration, *Rules and Regulations Governing Physicians' Services*, Official Bulletin No. 1246, April 24, 1940, p. 4.
33. Lee C. Dowling, "New York State's Public Medical Care Program," *New York State Journal of Medicine*, XLII (May 1, 1942), No. 9, 911.
34. Chicago Relief Administration, *Rules and Regulations Regarding Dental Care*. Official Bulletin No. 1255, May 3, 1940, pp. 3–4.
35. Robert S. Drews, "A History of the Care of the Sick Poor of the City of Detroit (1703–1855)," *Bulletin of the History of Medicine*, VII (July, 1939), No. 7, 765.
36. Grace W. Myers, *History of the Massachusetts General Hospital, June, 1872 to December, 1900*, Boston, 1929, p. 13. Quoted with permission of the publishers, Massachusetts General Hospital.
37. Joe Smith, *Kern General Hospital: 1867–1940*, Bakersfield, Cal., 1940, p. 12.
38. Department of Health for Scotland, Committee on Scottish Health Services, *Report*, Edinburgh, 1936, p. 213.
39. Chicago Relief Administration, *Rules and Regulations Governing Physicians' Services*, Official Bulletin No. 1246, April 24, 1940, p. 1.
40. State of Washington, *Session Laws of 1941*, Chap. 1, Par. 15.
41. State of Minnesota, *Session Laws of 1939*, Chap. 436, Sec. 12.
42. State of Michigan, *Public Acts 1941*, No. 343, Sec. 1.
43. U.S. Congress, Public Law 135, First Session, Seventy-eighth Congress, July 12, 1943.
44. Paul V. Benner, "Medical 'Insurance Plans' for Federal Assistance Cases in Kansas," *Medical Care*, III (May, 1943), 145–48.
45. Kansas State Department of Social Welfare, *Report of Social Welfare in Kansas*, No. 6, 1942, p. 18.
46. Margaret L. Plumley, "Out-Patient Operating Costs," *The Modern Hospital*, XLIX (Dec., 1937), No. 6, 65–67.
47. Harold S. Frum, *Choice and Change of Medical Service*, Committee on Research in Medical Economics, New York, 1939.

Gladys V. Swackhamer, *Choice and Change of Doctor*, Committee on Research in Medical Economics, New York, 1939.
48. Gertrude Sturges, "Home Medical Care," in Haven Emerson, ed., *Administrative Medicine*, New York, 1941, p. 153.
49. *Ibid.*, p. 142.
50. Ruth Houlton, "Public Health Nursing," *Social Work Year Book 1943*, New York, 1943, p. 401.
51. Dorothea M. Argo, "What Housekeeping Aides Do," *American Journal of Nursing*, XLI (July, 1941), No. 7, 775–80.
   Welfare Council of New York City, *Housekeeping Service for Chronic Patients*, mimeographed, 1942.
52. Franz Goldmann, "Hauspflege," in *Handbuch der Sozialen Hygiene und Gesundheitsfürsorge*, Berlin, 1927, VI, 229–69.
53. American Association of Medical Social Workers, *A Statement of Standards to Be Met by Medical Social Service Departments in Hospitals and Clinics*, rev. ed., Chicago, 1940, p. 3.
54. Margaret L. Plumley, *Medical Social Work in Tax-Supported Health and Welfare Services*, American Public Welfare Association, Chicago, 1940.
55. American Public Welfare Association, *Report of the Committee on Medical Care*, p. 39.
56. American Hospital Association and American Public Welfare Association, *Out-Patient Care for the Needy*, rev. ed., Chicago, 1942, pp. 11–12.
57. *Ibid.*, pp. 11–15.
58. Margaret L. Plumley, "Payments from Tax-Funds to Voluntary Hospitals for Out-Patient Service," *Hospitals*, XIV (Jan., 1940), No. 1, 99.
59. American Hospital Association, *Hospital Accounting and Statistics*, Chicago, 1937.
60. U.S. Children's Bureau, "Clinic Service—Instructions for Monthly Reports from Areas Cooperating in the Registration of Social Statistics, Form H-2, Social Statistics, Preliminary—January 1939."
61. Massachusetts Department of Public Welfare, *Manual of Public Assistance*, Chap. 10.
62. Henry Harris, *California's Medical Story*, Springfield, Ill., 1932, p. 113.
63. Grace W. Myers, *History of the Massachusetts General Hospital, June, 1872 to December 1900*, p. 140. Quoted with permission of the publishers, Massachusetts General Hospital.
64. Elliott H. Pennell and Joseph W. Mountin, "The Financial

Support of Non-Government Hospitals as Revealed by the Recent Federal Business Census of Hospitals," *Hospitals*, XI (Dec., 1937), No. 12, 14.
65. American Hospital Association and American Public Welfare Association, "Hospital Care for the Needy," *Hospitals*, XIII (Jan., 1939), No. 1, 23–25.
66. State of New York, *Session Laws of 1940*, Chap. 619, Art. 5, Title 4.
67. Marshall L. Pickens, "Payment by Local Authorities for the Care of Indigent Patients in General Hospitals," *Hospitals*, XVII (Jan., 1943), No. 1, 53.
68. State of Rhode Island, "Standard Hospital Agreement between Participating Hospitals, Rhode Island Local Departments of Public Welfare and the State Department of Social Welfare," Aug. 17, 1942.
69. Elliott H. Pennell and Joseph W. Mountin, "The Financial Support of Non-Government Hospitals as Revealed by the Recent Federal Business Census of Hospitals," *Hospitals*, XI (Dec., 1937), No. 12, 17.
70. Ernst P. Boas and Nicholas Michelson, *The Challenge of Chronic Diseases*, New York, 1929.
Ernst P. Boas, *The Unseen Plague—Chronic Disease*, New York, 1940.
71. Mary C. Jarrett, *Chronic Illness in New York City*, New York, 1933.
72. American Hospital Association and American Public Welfare Association, *Institutional Care of the Chronically Ill*, Chicago, 1940, p. 7.
73. E. M. Bluestone, "Chronic Disease—A Problem in Philanthropy," *Bulletin of the American Hospital Association*, IX (July 1935), No. 7, 55–64; and "Hospitals for Chronic Disease," in Haven Emerson, ed., *Administrative Medicine*, pp. 99–101.
74. "Chronic Disease Patients," *The Modern Hospital*, LIV (Jan., 1940), No. 1, 67–76.
75. American Hospital Association and American Public Welfare Association, *Institutional Care of the Chronically Ill*, p. 7.
76. N. I. Bowditch, *A History of the Massachusetts General Hospital*, Boston, 1872, p. 7.
77. State of New Jersey, Department of Institutions and Agencies, *Minimum Standards for Nursing Homes*, Trenton, 1941.
78. American Hospital Association and American Public Welfare Association, *Institutional Care of the Chronically Ill*, pp. 10–13.

79. State of Connecticut, *Report of the Commission to Study the Pauper Laws*, p. 5.
80. Michael M. Davis, *Public Medical Services*, Chicago, 1937, p. 146.
81. Quoted from the *Social Security Bulletin*, IV (Dec., 1941), No. 12, 1.
82. State of Connecticut, *Report of the Commission to Study the Pauper Laws*, p. 163.
83. Joseph W. Mountin and Evelyn Flook, "Distribution of Health Services in the Structure of State Government," Chap. VI, "Medical and Dental Care by State Agencies," *Public Health Reports*, LVII (Sept. 4, 1942), No. 36, 1248–52.
84. State of Rhode Island, *Public Laws of 1942*, Chap. 1212, Art. 1, Sec. 5.
85. State of North Dakota, *Session Laws of 1933*, Chap. 97, Sec. 5.
86. Michael M. Davis, *Public Medical Services*, p. 126.
87. American Public Welfare Association, *Organization and Administration of Tax-Supported Medical Care*, p. 6.
88. New York State Department of Social Welfare, *Medical Care Program for Locally Administered Medical Care Plans*, p. 1.
89. Nassau County Department of Public Welfare, *Manual of Medical Care*, Mineola, N.Y., 1942, p. 1.
90. State of Tennessee, *Public Acts 1939*, Chap. 102, title of act.
91. Joseph W. Mountin, "Administration of Public Medical Service by Health Departments," *American Journal of Public Health*, XXX (Feb., 1940), No. 2, 138.
92. New York State Department of Social Welfare, *Medical Care Program for Locally Administered Medical Care Plans*, p. 1.
93. State of Michigan, *Public Acts 1941*, Chap. 343, Sec. 1.
94. Information from the Indiana Department of Public Welfare.
95. Suffolk County Department of Public Welfare, *Manual of Medical Care*, Bayshore, N.Y., 1942, p. 7.
96. Nathan Sinai, Marguerite F. Hall, and Royden E. Holmes, *Medical Relief Administration*, Essex County Medical Economic Research, Windsor, Ontario, 1939.
97. *Ibid.*, p. 23. Quoted with permission of the publishers, Essex County Medical Economic Research.
98. Louis S. Reed and Dean A. Clark, "Appraising Public Medical Services," *American Journal of Public Health*, XXXI (May, 1941), No. 5, 421.
99. New Mexico Department of Public Welfare, *Survey of Medical Care and Health Status of Recipients of Public Assistance*, Santa Fé, 1944.

100. Nassau County Department of Public Welfare, *Public Assistance in 1942*, Fifth Annual Report, p. 33.
101. From unpublished studies by Dean A. Clark, M.D., and Louis S. Reed, Ph.D. Data used with permission of the U.S. Public Health Service.
102. Nathan Sinai, Marguerite F. Hall, V. M. Hogue, and Miriam Steep, *Medical Relief in Michigan*. Ann Arbor, 1938, p. 123.
103. From unpublished studies by Dean A. Clark, M.D., and Louis S. Reed, Ph.D. Data used with permission of the U.S. Public Health Service.
104. *Ibid.*
105. I. S. Falk and Anne E. Geddes, "Medical Care in Public Welfare Programs," *Medical Care*, I (Winter issue, 1941), No. 1, 73.

5: ADMINISTRATION OF PUBLIC MEDICAL CARE: ITS PRESENT FRAMEWORK

1. H. Jackson Davis, "Public Medical Care: Some Practical Considerations," *Connecticut State Medical Journal*, VII (Sept., 1943), No. 9, 623.
2. Joseph W. Mountin and Evelyn Flook, "Distribution of Health Services in the Structure of State Government," Chap. III, "Tuberculosis Control by State Agencies," *Public Health Reports*, LVII (Jan. 16, 1942), No. 3, 79.
3. Joseph W. Mountin and Evelyn Flook. "Distribution of Health Services in the Structure of State Government," Chap. VI, "Medical and Dental Care by State Agencies," *Public Health Reports*, LVII (Aug. 14, 1942), No. 33, 1196.
4. U.S. Children's Bureau, *Facts about Crippled Children*, Publication 293, Washington, D.C., 1942, p. 4.
5. American Public Welfare Association, Committee on Medical Care, *Cooperation in the Administration of Tax-Supported Medical Care*, Chicago, 1940, pp. 3–4.

6: PLANNING FOR MEDICAL CARE

1. First Inter-American Conference on Social Security, Sept. 10–16, 1942, "Declaration of Santiago de Chile," *Inter-American Committee on Social Security, Provisional Bulletin*, Aug., 1943, No. 3, cover page.
2. E. Wight Bakke, "The Debate on Socialized Medicine—A Layman's View," *Connecticut State Medical Journal*, VI (Oct., 1942), No. 10, 782. Quoted with permission of the publishers.

3. Arthur A. Ballantine, "The Situation Calls for Central Planning," *The Modern Hospital*, LX (June, 1943), No. 6, 86.
4. Hospital Council of Greater New York, *Use of Tax Funds to Pay for Care of the Indigent Sick in the Voluntary Hospitals of New York City*, New York, 1940, p. 18. Quoted with the permission of the Council.
5. Board of Trustees of the American Hospital Association, June 18, 1938, *Hospitals*, XII (July, 1938), No. 7, cover page. Quoted with permission of the American Hospital Association.
6. American Medical Association, Council on Medical Education and Hospitals, "Essentials of a Registered Hospital," *Journal of the American Medical Association*, CXII (May 27, 1939), No. 21, 2166.
7. Michael M. Davis, *America Organizes Medicine*, New York and London, 1941, p. 222.
8. Committee on the Costs of Medical Care, *Medical Care for the American People*, Chicago, 1932, pp. 109–18.
9. M. Sarraz-Bournet, "Esquisse d'une politique hospitalière," address before the first meeting of the Conseil Supérieur de l'Assistance Publique, Paris, Jan., 1932. Summary in "D'une organisation hospitalière rationelle, la hiérarchie dans les hôpitaux," *Nosokomeion*, V (1934), No. 1, 13–17.
10. British Medical Association, Medical Planning Commission, "Draft Interim Report," *British Medical Journal*, June 20, 1942, 745–46. Quoted with permission of the British Medical Association.
11. Medical Planning Research, "Interim General Report," Supplement to *The Lancet*, CCXLIII (Nov. 21, 1942), 599–622.
12. British Ministry of Health, *A National Health Service*, London, Feb., 1944, p. 15.
13. Commonwealth of Australia, National Health and Medical Research Council, *Report*, Twelfth Session, Canberra, 1941. Excerpt in *International Labour Review*, XLVII (June, 1943), No. 6, 733.
14. Kendall Emerson, "Responsibility of Organized Medicine in Medical Care," *American Journal of Public Health*, XXX (Oct., 1940), No. 10, 1174. Quoted with permission of the publishers.
15. Committee of Physicians for the Improvement of Medical Care, *Aims of the Committee*, March 4, 1940, p. 4.
16. Roger I. Lee and Lewis W. Jones, *The Fundamentals of Good Medical Care*, Publication No. 22 of the Committee on the Costs of Medical Care, Chicago, 1933, pp. 93–128.

17. Committee on the Costs of Medical Care, *Medical Care for the American People*, pp. 109 and 155. Quoted with permission of the publishers, The University of Chicago Press.
18. Editorial, *Journal of the American Medical Association*, XCIX (Dec., 1932), No. 23, 1950–52.
19. Committee of Physicians for the Improvement of Medical Care, *Principles and Proposals*, and subsequent statements.
20. British Ministry of Health, *Interim Report on the Future Provision of Medical and Allied Services* (Lord Dawson of Penn, Chairman), 1920.
21. British Medical Association, Medical Planning Commission, "Draft Interim Report," *British Medical Journal*, June 20, 1942, 749–50. Quoted with permission of the British Medical Association.
22. Medical Planning Research, "Interim General Report," Supplement to *The Lancet*, CCXLIII (Nov. 21, 1942), No. 6221, 618.
23. British Medical Association, Annual Representative Meeting 1943, Supplement to the *British Medical Journal*, Oct. 16, 1943, 69. Quoted with permission of the British Medical Association.
24. British Ministry of Health, *A National Health Service*, p. 28.
25. Commonwealth of Australia, National Health and Medical Research Council, *Report*, Twelfth Session, Canberra, 1941, as quoted in the *International Labour Review*, XLVII (June, 1943), No. 6, 734.
26. "Medical Planning," *The Medical Journal of Australia*, XXXI, (March 11, 1944), No. 11, 229.
27. Information from the New Zealand Legation, Washington, D.C.
28. Canadian House of Commons, Special Committee on Social Security, *Health Insurance: Report of the Advisory Committee on Health Insurance*, Ottawa, 1943, p. 23.
29. Helen Clapesattle, *The Doctors Mayo*, Minneapolis, Minn., 1941, p. 706.
30. Canadian House of Commons, Special Committee on Social Security, *Minutes of Proceedings and Evidence*, March 16, 1943, No. 1, 17.
31. Sir William Beveridge, *Social Insurance and Allied Services*, American ed., New York, 1942, p. 107.
32. Canadian House of Commons, Special Committee on Social Security, *Minutes of Proceedings and Evidence*, March 16, 1943, No. 1, 17.
33. Quoted from article "Insurance," the *Encyclopedia Britannica*, 14th ed., 1929, XII, 452–53.

34. Franz Goldmann, "Arbeitsgemeinschaften in der Gesundheitsfürsorge," in *Ergebnisse der Sozialen Hygiene und Gesundheitsfürsorge*, Leipzig, 1929, I, 264–90.
35. Commonwealth of Australia, National Health and Medical Research Council, *Report*, Twelfth Session, Canberra, 1941.
36. Department of Health for Scotland, Committee on Scottish Health Services, *Report*, Edinburgh, 1936, p. 168.
37. "Planning of Medical Care in the British Commonwealth of Nations," *Inter-American Committee on Social Security, Provisional Bulletin*, Oct., 1943, No. 4, 21.
38. R. O. Davison, "Municipal Medical Service in Saskatchewan," *Canadian Medical Association Journal*, XLV (Sept., 1941), 272–75.
39. British Ministry of Health, *A National Health Service*, p. 12.
40. U.S. Congress, H.R. 2861 and S. 1161, First Session, Seventy-eighth Congress, May 24, 1943.
41. U.S. Children's Bureau, *Memorandum to the States*, July 6, 1943.
42. U.S. Congress, H.R. 2861 and S. 1161, Sec. 14.
43. Medical Planning Research, "Interim General Report," Supplement to *The Lancet*, CCXLIII (Nov. 21, 1942), 613.
44. Franz Goldmann, "Instruction in Social and Economic Aspects of Medicine," *Journal of the Association of American Medical Colleges*, XVI (Sept., 1941), No. 5, 299–307.
45. British Ministry of Health, *A National Health Service*, p. 14.
46. U.S. Congress, H.R. 2861 and S. 1161, Sec. 11.
47. Samuel J. Rosenman, ed., *The Public Papers and Addresses of Franklin D. Roosevelt*, New York, 1938, I, pp. 351–52. Quoted with permission of the publishers, Random House, Inc.
48. Committee of Physicians for the Improvement of Medical Care, *Principles and Proposals*, p. 2.
49. U.S. Senate, *Preliminary Report from the Committee on Education and Labor on S. 1620*, First Session, Seventy-sixth Congress, Report No. 1139, Aug., 1939, p. 17.
50. National Resources Planning Board, *National Resources Development*. Part I, *Post-War Plan and Program*, H.R. Document No. 128, 1943, p. 3.
51. International Labor Conference, "Medical Care Recommendation, 1944 (No. 69)," Second Session, Seventy-eighth Congress, House Document No. 671, pp. 32–50.
52. Sir Arthur Newsholme, *Medicine and the State*, London and Baltimore, 1932, p. 29. Quoted with permission of the publishers, The Williams and Wilkins Company.

INDEX

Ability to pay, procedure for determining, 15, 48, 79-80
Adequacy of service, components of adequate program, 160; establishment and maintenance of, 139-47; necessity for annual reports: data needed, 145 ff.; professional supervision of, 140 ff.; wide spread between service provided and standards of adequacy, 147-148
Adirondack Cottage Sanitarium, 16
Administration, advisory committees, 138 f., 195; centralization or decentralization, 192-94; changes and improvements in organization, 129-50; coordination of medical care and social work, 186 f.; distribution of financial responsibility for public medical care, 153-55; establishment and maintenance of adequacy of service, 139-47; Federal responsibility, 21, 31, 41, 52, 60, 133; flaws in the administrative structure, 152 f.; framework of administrative structure: policies summarized, 151-57; health department vs. welfare department, 135-36; health insurance programs, 185; lack of trained administrators, 156; lay persons responsible for, 133-35; local responsibility, 21, 31, 35, 41, 50, 60, 129-38, 152-54; main categories of official agencies, 152; methods of assuring competence of personnel, 194 f.; multiplicity of agencies and practices, 131 f., 152-53; need for annual reports: statistical data for, 145 ff.; planning for the future administrative organization, 191-96; professional direction and supervision of programs, 138-88, 140 ff., 194-96; regional organization, 168, 193; standardization of public medical care, 155 f.; state responsibility, 21, 31, 41, 60, 131-33, 144, 154; training of administrators, 195; unification of local administration, 130, 136, 194
Administrators of medical care programs, 133-38, 140 ff., 194-96; training of, 195
Admission policies, clinics, 44, 48 f., 58 f., 116; hospitals: communicable disease, 11, 14 f., general, 37 ff., mental, 28-30, tuberculosis, 20, voluntary, 120 f.; policies of the past, 70-71; principles of temporary programs, 80, 120; see also Eligibility; Need
Advisory committees, 138 f., 195
Agricultural regions, see Rural areas
Aid to dependent children, see Dependent children
"All-out state medicine" and its implications, 180, 181; see also Government; Russia
Almshouses, conversion into chronic disease hospitals, 125; conversion into homes for the chronic sick, 128; early provisions for sick in, 9, 11, 24, 85 f., 87, 93; hospital units in, 127; trend from outdoor relief to care in, 85
Ambulance service, 128 f.
American Association of Medical Social Workers, 108
American College of Surgeons, 7, 33, 36, 37, 121; development of standards: for clinics, 46, for hospitals, 7, 38
American Hospital Association, 107, 116, 165; Committee on Hospital Planning and Equipment, 18; Committee on Out-Patient Work, 46, 49; on admission procedure for clinics, 48; on physicians' services in hospitals, text, 166-67; on service to the needy, 79
—— and American Public Welfare Association, joint committee, recommendations on institutional care, 120, 125, 128
American Medical Association, 11, 25, 82, 33, 86, 87, 89; attitude toward group practice, 66 f., 174; Council on Medical Education and Hospitals, 33; court ruling against, 67; Judicial Council, quoted, 66; on medical care for the needy, 77, 79
American Psychiatric Association, 27
American Public Health Association, Committee on Administrative Practice, 17
American Public Welfare Association, 80, 82, 88, 116, 185; "Essentials of Tax-Supported Medical Service," 83 f.; recommendations on: determination of eligibility, 80, professional direction of programs, 135
—— and American Hospital Association,

216 INDEX

American Public Welfare (*Continued*)
  joint committee, recommendations on institutional care, 120, 125, 128
American Sanatorium Association, 16
Analytical Chart of Reimbursable Medical, Dental and Nursing Care, N.Y., 133
Appliances, provision of, 113 f.
Application, as basis of service, 70, 78, 83, 180
Armed forces, Federal provision for, 69, 180; program for wives and infants of enlisted men, 78, 89, 96, 191
Assistance, public, beneficiaries as clinic clients, 48; divorce of health service from, 190; legal substitution of the principle of need, for destitution, 77; medical care recognized as "essential relief need," 75 ff.; new system substituted for outworn relief provisions, 73; three preferred groups of beneficiaries, 74; *see also* Relief
Atlantic Charter, 198
Attendants in mental hospitals, 27
Auburn, N.Y., 150
Australia, 65; planning, 169, 175, 176, 187, 188
Austria, 25, 31, 35

Bard, Samuel, 33
Beers, Clifford Whittingham, 27
Belgium, 22
Bellevue Hospital, 35 f., 107, 128
Beveridge, Sir William, quoted, 183
Bicêtre, the, 27
Blind, provision for, 74, 145, 155
Bloomingdale Hospital, 24
Boas, Ernst P., 125
Bodington, George, 16
"Body of Liberties . . . ," Massachusetts, 23
Bond, Thomas, 33
Boston, 14, 34, 57, 64, 93
Boston Almshouse, 36
Boston Dispensary, 45, 48
Bourgeois, Léon, 61
Brehmer, Hermann, 16
British Hospitals Association, 169
British Medical Association, 174; planning, 169, 175
——— in Australia, 65, 176, 186
Bruce, Isabel C., and Edith Eickhoff, 85
Budin, Pierre-Constant, 52
Buffalo, N.Y., 57
Bureau of Medical Economics, report quoted, 66
Byrnes, Justice, 131

California, 9, 24, 39, 57, 93
California Physicians' Service, 52
Canada, 143, 186, 188, 189
Canadian National Health Act, 176, 190
Cancer clinics, 60
Capitation system of paying physicians, 97, 100
Case work, medical social service as a branch of, 107, 108
Cash payment to the sick, for medical care expenses, 74, 190 f.
Census Bureau, U.S., 32, 162
Centralization or decentralization of administration, 192-94
Charité, La, 9
Chesterfield, Va., 150
Chicago Relief Administration, 90, 138; program of dental care, 91; *Rules . . . Governing Physicians' Services*, excerpt, 96
Children, aid to dependent, 74, 155; crippled, 81, 88, 140, 152, 153, 154 (*see entries under* Crippled); maternity and infant health services, 53, 60, 78, 86, 89, 96, 191; preventive clinics, 58, 60; school health services, 53, 55, 56, 60; well-baby services, 52, 55, 60
Children's Bureau, U.S., 116; quoted, 191
Chile, 52, 65
Chronic disease, custodial institutions, 126-28; housekeeping service, 106; visiting nurses' service, 105
——— hospitals, advantages and costs, 163; lack of facilities, 7, 123-24; provision of, and payment for, care of the needy in, 124-26
Cities, *see* Urban centers
Civil service, medicine under, 187
Clark, Dean A., and Louis S. Reed, 147
Clinics, admission policies, 44, 48 f., 58 f., 65, 67; basic objections to, 66, 103-4; charges and costs, 49-50, 59; classification of, 43 f., 52-53; departmentalization of treatment clinics, 46-47; determination of eligibility, 48-49, 59; district health center as outgrowth of, 57; educational value, 47, 54, 62; effect of preventive services on demand for treatment, 54; history, 44-45, 52, 62; income sources, 50, 51 f., 63, 115 f.; laboratories, 109, 110; medical social service in, 107, 108; number and distribution, 46, 53, 62; organization of care of the needy, 45 ff., 115-18; organization of physicians' services, 95, 102, 173 ff.; origin as dispensaries, 43, 44, 48; payment

INDEX

for services of nongovernmental clinics, 51, 116-17; preventive clinics, 47, 52-61; private group clinics, 43, 61-63, 65-67; problem of function of, in total program, 117, 169-70; public responsibility for provision of, 51, 60 f.; relationship between preventive and treatment services, 55, 67 f., 173 f.; relationship of nonprofit clinics to private physicians, 63-65; relative merits, 103-4; restriction or abolition of? 118; traveling clinics, 58; treatment clinics, 44-52, 81, 86, 103-4, 117-18; trend from limited to broad functions, 43, 45, 47, 51, 54 ff., 62, 67-68; unsolved problems, 67; utilization of hospital resources, 51, 56, 57, 173, 176-77

Collapse therapy, 18

Colonial and post-Revolutionary attitude toward, and provision for, the sick poor, 5, 8, 22 ff., 33, 70 f., 129, 131

Colonies, for tuberculous persons, 19

Committee of Physicians for the Improvement of Medical Care, 77, 174, 197

Committee on Research in Medical Economics, 174

Committee on the Costs of Medical Care, membership, 173; recommendations: on group practice, 167, 173, on hospital beds, 26

Committees, advisory, 138 f., 195

Committees, A.H.A., *see* American Hospital Association

Communicable disease hospitals, *see* Isolation hospitals

Community Facilities Act, 41

"Concerning the Relief of the Poor . . ." (Vivès), 72

Connecticut, 85, 130; mental defectives, 24

Consultant service, 175, 176

Contract practice, 66, 93

Convalescent homes, advantages and costs, 163; lack of facilities, 7, 123-24

Costs, *see* Financing; Volume and cost

Cottage hospital, 162

Council on Medical Education and Hospitals, 33

Crippled children, 81, 88; adequacy of service for, 140; agencies administering programs, 152, 153; Federal grants for programs, 154

Custodial care, defects in the past, 5; inadequate facilities, 123, 127; public provisions for, 126-28 (*see also* Chronic disease)

Davis, H. Jackson, 151

Davis, Michael M., 86, 174; quoted, 9, 130, 135, 167

Dawson Committee, 174

Dawson of Penn, Lord, quoted, 187

Decentralization or centralization of administration, 192-94

Declaration of Independence, 197

Demand for medical care, factors influencing, 171

Denmark, 19, 21, 41

Dental care program, Chicago, 91

Dentistry, clinics, 53, 55, 56, 58, 60

Dentists, advantages of health insurance programs, 185; costs of services to recipients of public assistance, 149; on mental hospital staffs, 27; organization of services, 92n; professional supervision, 142

Dependency, prevention of, an objective of medical care, 75; sickness as cause and result of, 72, 75

Dependent children, medical care for, 74, 155

Depressions, effects, 73, 120

Destitution, principle of need substituted for, in modern laws, 77; *see also* Need

Detroit, 85, 93, 134

Dettweiler, Peter, 16

Diagnosis, clinic service, 52, 54, 59; laboratory service, 109-11

Disease, recognition of mental deviation as, 23

Diseases, types of, in hospitals for communicable diseases, 11 ff.; *see also* under names, e.g., Tuberculosis; Venereal disease

Dispensaries, free, 43, 44 f., 48; *see also* Clinics

District health centers, 57; *see also* Planning, for group practice

District physician system, 95, 101 f.

Dix, Dorothea Lynde, 26

Drug dispensaries, 43, 44, 45, 48

Drugs, cost of, for recipients of public assistance, 149; organization of, and payment for, 111-13, 117, 121; problems presented, 112; supervisory procedures, 113; trend of pubic policy, 88

Duke Endowment, 122

Eastern State Hospital, 22

Economic need, *see* Need

Education, health guidance as function of the public health nurse, 105; medical, inadequately adjusted to new needs and

INDEX

Education (*Continued*)
opportunities, 156; training of specialists in administration, 195; value of clinics in training professional personnel, 47, 54, 62
Eickhoff, Edith, and Isabel C. Bruce, 85
Eligibility for public medical care, determination of, by untrained persons, 134; economic need as basis for, 15, 20, 30, 38 f., 48, 58 f., 77 ff., 180-81, 188; groups eligible, 69; procedure under modern programs, 79 f.; regardless of income or residence, 69, 78, 180; standards of, liberalized, 78-82; *see also* Admission; Need
Elizabethan Poor Law Act, 14, 36, 70; *see also* Poor Laws
Emergency maternity and infant care, 89, 96, 191
Emerson, Haven, quoted, 57
Emerson, Kendall, quoted, 169
England, *see* Great Britain
Enlisted men, *see* Armed forces
"Essentials of Tax-Supported Medical Service," 83 f.
Essex County Hospital for Contagious Diseases, Belleville, N.J., 12
Ethics, medical: statements by American Medical Association, 66
Eye diseases and defects, 58, 60
Eyeglasses, provision of, 113 f.

Farm Security Administration, 51
Federal Emergency Relief Administration, program, 75, 133
Federal Emergency Relief Administration Act, 86, 95
Federal government, *see* Government
Federal hospitals, *see subdivisions under* Hospitals
Fee-for-service method of payment, 63, 66, 97, 100 f., 141, 142, 143
Fees of clinic patients, 49 f.
"Fever hospitals," 9, 11, 14
Financing public medical care, clinic care, 51, 116-17; distribution of responsibility: trends summarized, 153-55; Federal-state cooperation, 41, 60, 133, 154 f., 191; general hospital care, 34, 39, 118-23; hospitalization for: communicable diseases, 15, mental illness, 29-30, tuberculosis, 20-22; state-local cooperation, 78, 131-33, 154; *see also* Payment methods
Foreign governments, *see under* Government; National

Forlanini, Carlo, 19
France, 9, 22, 25, 27, 31, 41, 161, 168; clinics, 52, 61, 65, 67; public aid declared duty in her Constitution, 197
Franklin, Benjamin, quoted, 83
Freeborn County, Minn., 150
Free-choice principle, 94, 95, 97, 99 f., 113, 141, 142, 143, 177 f., 187
Free dispensaries, 43, 44 f., 48; *see also* Clinics
Freedman's Hospital, 36
"Freedom of choice of vendor," 113
Full-time physicians, 7, 27, 51, 63, 95, 98, 102, 135 ff., 181, 186-88, 194
Fundamentals of Good Medical Care, The (Lee and Jones), 171

General hospitals, administrative responsibility for public facilities, 35, 37, 41, 131, 152-53; admission policies, 37 ff., 120; communicable disease units, 13, 162; cost of services to recipients of public assistance, 149; extent of hospitalization, 39; functional coordination of general and special hospitals, 168; function in the community health program, 166 f.; growth: statistics, 32, 37; inclusive rates of payment and per diem rates, 121; income from tax funds, 40, 119, 122-23; mental disease units, 24, 26, 162; organization of care of the needy in, 113-24; organization of physicians' services, 7, 95, 98 (*see* Physicians); payment of tax funds to nongovernmental facilities, 118-22, 182; policies followed by various countries in providing for, 31, 39, 41, 186; problem of proper utilization, 123; procedure in hospitalization of the individual, 122; public responsibility for establishment of, 4, 31-42; quality of facilities, 33; role of nonprofit voluntary and proprietary facilities, 34, 42, 121; tuberculosis units, 17, 18, 20, 162; undersupply of facilities, 33; use of tax funds, 120 ff. (*see* Taxes; Payment methods); utilization of nongovernmental facilities, 120 f., 165-66, 182, 185, 188; voluntary effort: pioneers in the field, 83 ff.
General Public Assistance Act, R.I., 77, 132
Germany, 14, 31, 65, 81, 161, 186; mental hospitals, 30; public assistance law, 73; tuberculosis hospitals, 16, 19
Gonorrhea, 12, 81; *see also* Venereal disease

INDEX

Government, "all-out state medicine" and its implications, 180-81; extent of public responsibility for establishment of clinics, 51, 60, of hospitals: communicable disease, 11, 14, general, 35, 37, mental, 26, tuberculosis, 21; extent of public responsibility for payment of care in governmental general hospitals, 37, 40, in governmental mental hospitals, 29-31, in nongovernmental clinics, 116, in nongovernmental hospitals, 21, 122 f., in public tuberculosis hospitals, 21; Federal reimbursement of state expenditures: statistics, 154 f.; Federal-state cooperation, 52, 60 f., 104, 133, 154 f., 191; principle of public responsibility for support of clinics, 43, 50, 51, 59, 115 f., of hospitals, 165 f., of communicable disease facilities, 8 f., 11, of general hospitals, 81, 34-36, 38 f., 41, of mental hospitals, 22, of tuberculosis hospitals, 20; public responsibility for payment of care in nongovernmental clinics, 116, in nongovernmental hospitals, 119 ff.; public responsibility for hospitals in various foreign countries, 8, 11, 14, 15, 19 f., 21 f., 26, 30 f., 39, 40 f., 186; "right to health service," 75, 186 ff., 196-98; self-supporting groups that are beneficiaries of Federal provisions, 69; *see also* Administration

Gradualism, policy of, and its effects, 188

Grants-in-aid, basis of allotment, 155; role in health policy, 154

Grasslands Hospital, 36

Great Britain, clinics, 52, 61, 64, 65; communicable disease hospitals, 11, 14; early social philosophy *re* care of the needy, 5, 70, 71, 72; general hospitals, 31, 35, 36, 39, 41; health centers, 54, 174 f.; maternal and child health services, 60; mental hospitals, 23, 26, 28, 29, 30; new system of public assistance, 73, 74, 80, 81; planning, 168 f., 174, 175, 184, 187, 189, 195; school health service, 55; tuberculosis hospitals, 16, 19, 20, 22

Grey, Lord, Commission, 70

Group clinics, private, 43, 61-63, 65-67

Group Health Association, Washington, 67

Group practice, American Medical Association's stand, 67; conditions necessitating, 62; defined, 61; feasibility of, 176; free-choice principle, as related to, 177-78; income of physicians, 63; in foreign countries, 52, 174-76; opposition to, 66, 173-74; organization of, 62-63, 176 f.; proposals for generalization and views advocating and opposing, 173-78

Handicapped, medical care for, 81; *see also* Blind; Crippled children

Hartford Dispensary, 50

Harvard College, 98

Health centers, 57; in Great Britain, 54, 174 f.; in relation to group practice, 173 ff.; in Russia, 52; location, etc., 176; *see also* Clinics

Health conservation declared both right and obligation of state, 186 ff., 196-98

Health insurance, *see* Insurance

Health policies, inadequacy of earliest, 70-73; new system substituted, 78 ff.; philosophy underlying, 196-98

Health professions, *see* Professional personnel

Health Service, Public, U.S., 11, 59, 148

Health services, attitude of public health departments toward responsibility for medical care, 136, 196; divorce from public assistance, 190; Federal participation, 52, 60, 104, 133, 154 f., 191; hospital's function in health program, 167; laboratories, 109 f.; need for coordination of preventive and treatment services, 156; participation of all groups concerned in planning and operating, 195; public health nursing, 104-7, 109; public health objectives defined, 54

Home care, early "outdoor relief," 85; housekeeping service included in, 106; modern programs, 86 ff.; organization of physicians' service, 94 ff., 99-102; responsibility of clinics for, 44, 117, 118; visiting nurses' service included in, 88, 104 ff.

Hospital Council of Greater New York, quoted, 166

Hospitals, concepts of hospital and its objectives, 5-6; demand for hospitalization, 163-65; development of medical social service, 107, 108; from outdoor relief to hospitalization, 85; laboratory services, 109 f.; need for coordination and planning, 42; planning for hospitals and related facilities: points on which decisions necessary, 160-70; procedures for hospitalization and for controlling length of stay, 144; qualitative standards: necessary policies, 165; quantitative standards: factors to be

220   INDEX

Hospitals (*Continued*)
  considered, 163-65; regional organization, 168, 193; responsibility for provision of hospitals and related facilities, 165 f. (*see also* Government); specialization, degree of, 162 f.; the large and the small facility, 161 f.; utilization for clinic care, 51, 56, 57; variety of public agencies administering, 153
  —— chronic disease, *see* Chronic disease hospitals
  —— general, *see* General hospitals
  —— isolation, *see* Isolation hospitals
  —— mental, *see* Mental hospitals
  —— proprietary, *see* Voluntary hospitals
  —— public, facilities: for communicable diseases, 8-15, for mental deviations, 4, 22-31, for tuberculosis, 4, 16-22; general hospitals, 4, 31-42; growth, 4-42; lack of nation-wide hospital policy, 41; services available to all in foreign countries, 31, 39; statistics on total facilities and those for selected groups, 4; *see also* Government
  —— special, departmentalization, 7; functional coordination of special and general hospitals, 167; necessity of, 162 f.; *see also* Chronic disease hospitals; Convalescent homes
  —— tuberculosis, *see* Tuberculosis hospitals
  —— voluntary, *see* Voluntary hospitals
Hôtel Dieu, 25
Housekeepers, visiting, 106
Housing authorities, local, 51

Illness as cause and result of want, 72
Immunization, as clinic function, 47, 53, 60
Incomes, family, 76; group clinic physicians', 63
Indiana, 95; committee on medical aid, 139
Industrial workers, clinics for, 45, 49, 50, 53, 65
Infants, *see* Children
Insane, term, 22, 23
Institutional care, trend from outdoor relief to, 85; *see also* Hospitals
Institutions of almshouse type, *see* Almshouses
Insurance, administration of insurance programs, 185; advantages and limitations, 184 f.; compulsory health insurance *vs.* public medical care, 186-90; defined, 182; effect of health insurance on health professions and hospitals, 185; funds used for establishment of hospitals, 81, 188; principle applied to payment for care at clinics, 51; provisions of Wagner-Murray-Dingell Bill of 1943, 190
"Integrated acute-chronic hospital plan," 126
International Labor Conference, Medical Care Recommendation, 198
Ireland, clinics, 117; medical relief, 71
Isolation hospitals, 8-15, 162; admission policies of public hospitals, 11, 14; financing of care, 15; hospitalization should be available for everybody, 14, 15; liberal standards governing eligibility for medical care, 80; main types of facilities, 10; new phase of development in prevention and care, 9; policy in foreign countries, 10 f.; protection of the public *vs.* welfare of the patient, 9, 15; types of disease hospitalized, 12; units in general and special hospitals, 13, 162
Isolation of the infectious sick, 8 ff.; *see also* Isolation hospitals
Italy, tuberculosis hospitals, 19

Jackson, James, 127
Jacobs, Philip P., quoted, 17
Jail, mental patients in, 23, 24
Jarrett, Mary C., 125
Jones, Lewis W., and Roger I. Lee, 171
Journal of the American Medical Association, excerpt, 174
Judicial Council, A.M.A., quoted, 66
Justice Department, U.S., 67

Kansas, 98, 130
Kempf, Grover A., 29
Kern County, Calif., 9, 93
Koch, Robert, 19

Laboratory services, 109-11, 117, 121
Lancet, The, 35; excerpt, 64
Lay control, of medical care programs, 133-35
Lee, Roger I., and Lewis W. Jones, 171
Léon Bourgeois law of 1916, 61
License to practice medicine, need for nation-wide, 173
Licensing of facilities for the sick, 46, 165
Local Government Act, British, 22, 26, 39, 73 f.
Localities, administrative responsibilities of, 129 ff., 131 f., 152-54; responsibility

for clinics, 50, 60, for hospitals: communicable disease, 11, general, 35, 41, mental, 31, tuberculosis, 21; state-local cooperation in financing medical care, 132, 154; state supervisory control over, 141, 144; *see also* Administration

Louisiana, 38, 41

Low-income groups, recognition of need of, for medical care, 75 ff.

Luce, H. A., quoted, 79

Lunacy, term, 22, 23

Marine hospitals, 85

Maritime quarantine, 8

Massachusetts, 21, 23, 26, 29, 38, 78, 151

Massachusetts General Hospital, 34, 64, 120

Massachusetts *Manual of Public Assistance*, excerpt, 118

Maternity and infant health services, 53, 60, 78, 86, 89, 96, 191

Mayo, W. J., quoted, 178

Means test, 70, 83, 180

Medical Administration Service, 174

Medical Care Program . . . , N.Y., excerpt, 187

Medical care, public, defined, 1; development of programs for persons in need, 69-150 (*see entries under* Programs); development of public clinics, 43-61; development of public hospitals, 4-42; summary of directions of advance, 103

"Medical Care Recommendation" by International Labor Conference, 198

Medical centers, *see* Clinics and Health centers

"Medically needy," defined, 79 f.; development of medical care programs for the, 76-83

Medical Planning Commission, British, 174

Medical Planning Research, quoted, 174, 193

Medical Relief Charities Act, Ireland, 71, 117

Medical social service, 5, 27, 88, 107-9; coordination with physicians' service, 137; planning for, 170-73; relationship to public health nursing, 109

Mental clinics, 53, 60

Mental deviations, early provisions for, 23 f.; modern concepts, 23; old concepts, 22 f.; psychiatric services in general hospitals, 26, 163

Mental Diseases Act, Sweden, 29

Mental hospitals, 22-31; development and number of specialized services, 25 f.; functions of modern hospitals, 28; hospital facilities, 4, 162, 163; hospital population, 29; income from tax funds, 30, 123; policies governing admission to public hospitals, 28-30; professional personnel on staffs, 27; public responsibility for hospitals, 22, 26-31; types of facilities in modern programs, 25

Merit system, appointments on basis of, 102, 170, 187, 194

Metropolitan Asylum Board, 14

Michigan, 24, 85, 138, 148; laws *re* handicapped persons, 81; law *re* physicians' services, excerpt, 96

Milwaukee, Wis., 34

Minnesota, free choice, 96; law *re* communicable diseases, 15; volume and cost of medical care, 148-50

Mississippi, 41

Model Health Centre, British, plan of, 174

Montclair, N.J., 50

Mountainside Hospital, 49

Mountin, Joseph W., quoted, 136

Nassau County, N.Y., 136, 147

National Association for the Campaign against Tuberculosis in Sweden, 58

National Formulary, The, 113

National governments, need for participation in provision of hospitals, 21, 31, 40; participation of foreign governments in support of health facilities, 15, 21 f., 26, 30, 41, 60 f.; responsibility assumed by Federal government, 4; *see also* Government

National Health and Medical Research Council, Australia, 169, 175, 187; quoted, 176

National Health Inventory, 46

National Health Service, British, 175, 189, 195

National Resources Planning Board, 198

National Tuberculosis Association, 16, 59

"Necessary" medical care, determination of, 90

Need, economic, as basis of eligibility, 15, 20, 30, 38 f., 48, 58 f., 77 ff., 180 f., 188 (*see also* Admission); destitution alone recognized as prerequisite for community action, 35; evaluation of "medical need," 79; person in need, defined, 78, 79; principle of, substituted for destitution, in law, 77 f.; *see also* Eligibility for public medical care

Need for a National Health Program, The, 17, 26, 82
Needy, development of programs for medical care of, 69-150; *see entries under* Programs
New Haven Hospital, 50
New Jersey, 128
New Mexico, 147
Newsholme, Sir Arthur, quoted, 198
New York (city), early hospitals, 33, 35; health centers, 57; study of chronic illness in, 125
New York (state), colonial quarantine, 8; Department of Social Welfare, 90, 133; law re hospitalization, 121; *Medical Care Program . . . ,* excerpt, 137; professional direction of administration, 136; "Regulations Governing Medical Care in the Home . . . ," 86; Social Welfare Law, 77, 121; types of medical care that may be provided, list, 90 f.
New York Dispensary, 44
New York Hospital, 24
New Zealand, 26, 168, 176
North Carolina, 122
North Dakota, 134, 150
Northwest Territory, Australia, 134
Norway, 19, 21, 61
Nuffield Provincial Hospitals Trust, 169
Nuremberg, Ger., 14
Nurses, in mental hospitals, 27; public health nurses, 104 ff., 194; relationship between public health nursing and medical social work, 109; school for, at Bellevue, 36; service to recipients of public assistance: costs, 149; supervisory work, 142
Nursing homes, private, 125, 127 f.

Oakland County Contagious Hospital, Pontiac, Mich., 12
Occupational therapists, 27
Old age, "homes," 128; mental disorders, 28
Old-age assistance, 74, 155; medical care for recipients: statistics, 148, 149; *see also* Senior Citizens Grants Act
Ophthalmologist, supervising, 145
Orthopedic clinics, 53, 55, 56, 60
Outdoor relief, 85
Out-patient departments, 44 ff., 115 ff.; *see* Clinics
Overseers of the poor, 70, 134

Panel system, 94, 97, 99 f.
Paris hospitals, 9, 27

Paupers, colonial attitude toward, and care of, 70 f.; responsibility for nonresidents, 130, 131
Payment methods, insurance principle, 182-86; taxation principle, 179-82; use of insurance and taxation in combination vs. use of single method, 186-90; *see also* Financing public medical care
"Pay" patients, accepted by public hospitals, 15, 20, 30, 38; refused, 38 f.
Pennsylvania, 134; state responsibility for general hospitals, 41
Pennsylvania Hospital, Philadelphia, 24, 33
"Per diem method of payment," 121
Personnel, *see* Professional personnel
Peru, 52, 65
"Per-visit method of payment for clinic service," 116
Pesthouses, 11, 35
Peters, John P., 174
Pharmacists, provision of drugs and other supplies, 111, 112; supervisory work, 140
Philadelphia, early hospitals, 24, 33, 36
Philadelphia Dispensary, 44
Philadelphia General Hospital, 36
Philadelphia Hospital for Contagious Diseases, 11, 12
Philip, Sir Robert, 52
Philosophy, *see* Social philosophy
Physically handicapped, care for, 81; *see also* Blind; Crippled children
Physicians, advantages of health insurance programs, 185; attitude toward clinics in general, 118, toward group practice, 65-67, 173-74, 177, toward hospitals "practicing medicine," 166-67, toward nonprofit clinics, 63-65, toward state medicine, 187 f.; contract practice, 66, 93; cost of services to recipients of public assistance, 149; direction of medical care programs, 135-38, 156, 194-96; effect of scientific advance upon practice, 62, 158, 171 f.; exploitation by public agencies, 93; free choice of, 94, 95, 97, 99 f., 113, 141, 142, 143, 177 f., 187; group practice, 63 ff., 173-78; health departments headed by, 156; hospital policies re services, 7, 95, 98, 167, 170; inconsistencies in policies of public agencies, 98; methods of organizing and paying for services of, 92-104; participation in planning and operating programs, 138 f., 195; payment for services lacking, 86, 93, 98; private group

clinics, 43, 61-63, 65-67; ratio to population, 171 f.; relative merits of the various methods of organization and payment, 99-104; services in nonprofit clinics, 48, 58, 63-67, 95, 102 f.; services now more frequently available at public expense, 87; standards of competence, 102, 170, 194; supervision of own field, 142 ff.; *see also entries under* Professional

Pinel, Philippe, 27

Pioneer Health Centre at Peckham, 54

Pitié, La, 9

Planning: for administration of medical care, 191-96; for group practice, 173-78; for hospitals and related facilities, 160-70; for medical social service, 108; for organization of professional services, 170-78; for payment for facilities and services, 178-91; nation-wide and state-wide, increasing, 156; objectives of, 159-60; philosophy underlying, 196-98; scope of, 159-60

Pneumothorax, artificial, 19

Political influence, 134 f., 181, 187

Poor, the, *see* Need; Needy

Poorhouses, *see* Almshouses

Poor Law Act, British, 14, 36, 70

Poor Laws, gradual abandonment of, 71, 73, 74, 81, 83

Poor relief, *see* Relief

Prepayment method, 51, 63, 98, 182-85, 189-90

Prevention, distinction between treatment and, 55; need for unification of administration of preventive services and medical care, 156; prevention of dependency because of illness, a fundamental of public assistance policies, 75; principle violated by operating medical care programs on basis of application and eligibility requirements, 181; utilization of the general hospital for, 167

Preventive clinics, 43, 47, 52-61

Principles of Medical Ethics, A.M.A., excerpt, 66

"Procedural Instructions," New York . . . , 90

Professional direction of public medical care programs, 133-38, 156, 194-96; divisions of medical care in welfare departments, 135 ff. *passim;* duties of medical administrators in welfare departments, 137; supervision of professional matters as feature of newer policy, 140 ff.; *see also* Advisory committees

Professional personnel, appointments on basis of a merit system, 102, 187, 194; better distribution of, 172-78; competence of, 170, 194 f.; full-time salaried system: advantages and disadvantages, 187 f.; group practice, 61-63, 173-78; hospital staffs, 7, 27, 170; ratio to population, 172-78; *see also under group names, e.g.,* Dentists; Physicians; etc.

Professional services, laboratory service, 109-11; medical social service, 107-9; organization of, and payment for, 92-114; physicians' service, 92-104; planning for organization of, 170-78; provision of drugs and appliances, 111-18 f.; visiting nurses' service, 104-7

Programs of public medical care for the needy, adequacy of service, 139-47; administrative organization, 129-50; advisory committees, 138 f., 195; development of, 69-150; distribution of administrative responsibility, 129-33, 152-54; extension and improvement of services, 85-91; groups eligible for care, 69 (*see also* Admission; Eligibility); organization of, and payment for: care in chronic disease hospitals and custodial institutions, 124-29, clinic care, 115-18, general hospital care, 118-24, institutional care, 114-29; organization of, and payment for: ambulance service, 128 f., drugs and appliances, 111-14, laboratory service, 109-11, medical social service, 107-9, physicians' (and dentists') service, 92-104, visiting nurses' service, 104-7; professional direction, 133-38; public responsibility: from the "paupers" to the "medically needy," 70-83; role of American Public Welfare Association, 83: its "Essentials of . . . Medical Service," 83 f.; scope and components of adequate program, 84, 160; volume and cost of service, 147-50

Proprietary hospitals, *see* Voluntary hospitals

Psychologists, 27

Psychometrists, 27

Public assistance, *see* Assistance

Public health, *see* Health

Public health nurses, 104-7, 109, 194

Public Hospital for Persons of Insane and Disordered Mind, Virginia, 22

Public hospitals, *see* Hospitals, public

Public medical care, *see* Government; Medical care
Public Works Administration funds, 41

Quarantine, 8
Quincy City Hospital, 38

Reed, Louis S., and Dean A. Clark, 147
Regional organization, 168 f., 193
"Regulations Governing Medical Care in the Home . . . ," N.Y., 86
Relief, divorce of health service from, 190; evils of system, 72; expenditures for medical care of relief recipients, 148-50; medical care recognized as an essential relief need, 75; reorientation of public policy, 73 ff.; *see also* Assistance, public
Repayment for services, 180
Research, in clinics, 47; in group clinics, 62; in hospitals, 6, 161
Residence and settlement requirement, 14, 71, 83, 130, 190
Rhode Island, General Public Assistance Act, 77, 132; reimbursement of localities, 132; "Standard Hospital Agreement," 122
Roberts, Kingsley, 174
Rochester, N.Y., clinics, 47, 50
Rochester Hospital Council, 50
Roentgen, Wilhelm, 20
Roentgenological laboratories, 58, 109, 110
Roosevelt, Franklin Delano, quoted, 196
"Rotating panel," 94
Rowe, G. H. M., quoted, 14
Rules and Regulations Governing Physicians' Services, Chicago, excerpt, 96
Rural areas, action necessary to remedy undersupply of health personnel, 172-73; limitations of group practice, 176; potential advantages of full-time salaried service, 188; scarcity of clinics, 53, of general hospitals, 32, 37, of laboratories, 110, of nurses, 105
Russia, clinics, 52; hospitals, 31; state medical services for all, 186; venereal disease control program, 81

Sanatoria, tuberculosis, 16, 17, 18; *see also* Tuberculosis hospitals
San Francisco, 119
Saranac Lake, sanitarium at, 16
Sarraz-Bournet, M., plan for hospitals, 168
Scandinavian countries, 31, 81

Schlegel, G. W. F., quoted, 28
School health services, 53, 55, 56, 60
Scientific medicine, rise of, effect on practice of medicine and costs of medical care, 62, 158, 171-72
Scotland, 169
Self-supporting persons, median family income, 76; recognition of need for medical care, 75 ff.
Senate subcommittee, statement on health as a public concern, 197
Senile disorders, 28
Senior Citizens Grants Act, Washington, 74, 88
Service men, *see* Armed forces
Settlement and residence requirement, 14, 71, 83, 131, 190
Sisters of Charity . . . , Milwaukee, 34
Sisters of Mercy, San Francisco, 119
Smallpox, 8, 9, 10, 14
Social insurance, administration, 185 f.; effect on health professions and voluntary hospitals, 185; qualities and advantages, 184; relationship to public assistance and public medical care, 189; utilization for establishment of hospitals, 31; *see also* Insurance; Wagner-Murray-Dingell Bill of 1943
Social philosophy, 5, 14, 20 f., 22 f., 31, 35, 38, 51, 59 f., 70 ff., 81, 89 f., 114 f.; underlying modern health policy, 196-98
Social Security Act, 60, 73, 82, 104, 125, 133; Amendments of 1943, 190; financing of health services under terms of, 154 f.
Social Security Board, 145
Social service, medical, 5, 27, 88, 107-9, 137, 173
Social welfare, reorientation and expansion of public responsibility for, 73 ff.; *see also* Welfare departments
Social Welfare Department, N.Y., 90, 133
Social Welfare Law, N.Y., 77, 121
Social work, attempt to bring into close relation with preventive health activities, 54; coordination of medical care and, 137
Social workers, medical, 5, 27, 88, 107-9, 137, 142, 173
Socio-economic setting of illness, research in, 47
South America, 31, 52, 65
South Carolina, 35, 122
Special hospitals, *see* Hospitals, special
Specialists, fees, 97; in clinics, 103; in group practice plans, 176; in private

group clinics, 63; reluctant to serve under public programs, 99 ff.; services made available under modern programs, 87 ff.; standards for certification established, 170; training for administrative work, 195; *see also* Physicians
Spital zu St. Marx, 25
Standard Hospital Agreement, R.I., 122
State, the, *see* Government
States, administrative functions and powers, 131 f.; advisory committees, 139; Federal-state cooperation, 52, 60 f., 104, 133, 154 f., 191; laws *re* organization of physicians' services, 96; payment for services to wives and infants of enlisted men, 89; programs directed by physicians, 137; reimbursement of localities, 132; responsibility for general hospitals, 41, for mental hospitals, 31, for tuberculosis hospitals, 21; state-local cooperation for development of medical care programs, 132, 154, for development of preventive health services, 60, 154; "state paupers," 71; supervision of local programs, 141, 144; *see also* Administration; Government
Students, clinics for, 45, 49, 50, 53, 65
Suffolk County, N.Y., 141
Sumner, William Graham, quoted, 76
Supreme Court, U.S., ruling quoted, 67
Surgical methods in treatment of tuberculosis, 18
Sweden, clinics, 58, 61; communicable disease hospitals, 11, 15; general hospitals, 40, 41, 161, 162; mental hospitals, 29, 30; tuberculosis hospitals, 21; venereal disease control, 61
Switzerland, 22
Syphilis, 10, 12, 14, 81; *see also* Venereal disease

Taxes, combination of insurance and taxation, 51, 188-90; income source of nongovernmental clinics, 116, of nongovernmental hospitals, 21, 122, 123, of public clinics, 51, of public general hospitals, 40, of public mental hospitals, 30, of public tuberculosis hospitals, 21; method of taxation, its characteristics and potential application, 179-82, 186-89; use of tax funds to pay nongovernmental facilities, 115
Teaching opportunities in clinics, 47, 54, 62
Tennessee, 90, 136
Tennessee Valley Authority, 52

Township responsibility, principle of, 129
Transportation, 128 f.
Traveling clinics, 58
Treatment, distinction between prevention and, 55
Treatment clinics, 43, 44-52, 81, 86, 103-4, 117-18
Trudeau, Edward L., 16
Tubercle bacillus, 19
Tuberculosis Clinic Manual, 59
Tuberculosis clinics, 52, 53, 55, 58, 59, 60, 61; French law *re* clinics, 61
Tuberculosis hospitals, 16-22; admission policy of public hospitals, 20; functions of various facilities, 17-18; income of nongovernmental hospitals from tax funds, 123, of public hospitals, 21; public responsibility for support of, 4, 20-22; units in general or special hospitals, 11, 12, 17, 18, 20, 162 f.
Twain, Mark, 72

United States, clinics, 52, 53, 60, 62, 65, 66, 67, 118; compulsory health insurance proposed, 189-90; group practice proposed, 173 f.; groups to whom public medical care is available, 69, 75; need for over-all planning of hospitals, 42; number of aged, children, and blind aided, 74; policy *re* communicable disease hospitals, 8, 11, 12 ff., *re* general hospitals, 31-42 *passim*, 161, 162, *re* mental hospitals, 23 f., 26, 28, 29, 30, 31, *re* tuberculosis hospitals, 16, 17, 20, 21; public assistance, 73, 74, 86, 190; public hospitals, statistics, 4; tax money spent on medical care, 180; venereal disease control, 81; *see also* Government
United States Pharmacopœia, The, 113
United States Public Health Service, 11, 59, 148
University students, clinics for, 45, 49, 50, 53, 65
Urban centers, concentration of clinics, 53, of general hospitals, 32, 37, of laboratories, 110, of public health nurses, 105; group practice, feasibility, 176; suggested remedies for uneven distribution of health personnel, 172-73

Vaccination in clinics, 47, 53
Valhalla, N.Y., hospital, 36
Venereal disease, 11, 12, 162, 163; clinics, 53, 55, 58, 59, 60, 61; European control programs, 61, 81; Federal grants, 154; nation-wide control program, 81

Venereal Disease Control Act, 60
Veterans, 35, 69
Vienna, 25, 85
Village settlements for tuberculous patients, 19
Virchow, Rudolf, quoted, 6
Virginia, hospital for the mentally ill, 22; volume and cost of medical care, 149, 150
"Visit," clinic, defined, 116
Visiting housekeeper service, 106
Visiting nurses' service, 104-7
Vivès, Juan-Luis, quoted, 36, 72
Vocational Rehabilitation Act, 82
Volume and cost of service to persons in need, experiences illustrating, 147-50
Voluntary effort credited with development of clinics, 50, 59, of hospitals, 19, 88
Voluntary hospitals, future, 42, 165-66; income from tax funds, 21, 119 ff., 122 f.; leaders in the field, 19, 33; number of general hospitals, 34, of isolation hospitals, 11, of mental hospitals, 26, of tuberculosis hospitals, 20; payment for care of the needy, 118-22; role in community, 88; supervision by the state? 81
Voluntary Hospitals Commission, British, 169
Voluntary Hospitals Committee, British, 168

Wagner Bill of 1939, 197
Wagner-Murray-Dingell Bill of 1943, 174, 190, 191, 195
Wales, 56, 60
Warren, John C., 127
Washington, D.C., 36, 57, 67
Washington, state, 74, 88, 96; State-Medical-Dental Board, 139
Welfare departments, advisory committees, 138 f.; attitude toward responsibility for general medical care, 136; divisions of medical care, 135; duties of medical director, 137; medical care expenditures, 148-50; see also Social welfare
Well-baby conference, 52; clinics, 55, 60
Wells, H. G., 198
Whittemore, James H., quoted, 64
Wilkes-Barre, Pa., 57
Williams, J. H. Harley, quoted, 5
Winslow, C.-E. A., quoted, 54
Wives and infants of enlisted men, 78, 89, 96, 191
Workhouses, see Almshouses
Works Progress Administration, 41, 82, 106

X ray, discovery of, 20; examinations, 58; laboratories, 109, 110

Yale School of Medicine, 50

Bei Fragen zur Produktsicherheit wenden Sie sich bitte an:
If you have any questions regarding product safety,
please contact:

Walter de Gruyter GmbH
Genthiner Straße 13
10785 Berlin
productsafety@degruyterbrill.com